UNCERTAINTY IN MEDICINE

UNCERTAINTY IN MEDICINE

A Framework for Tolerance

Paul K.J. Han

OXFORD
UNIVERSITY PRESS

OXFORD
UNIVERSITY PRESS

Oxford University Press is a department of the University of Oxford. It furthers
the University's objective of excellence in research, scholarship, and education
by publishing worldwide. Oxford is a registered trade mark of Oxford University
Press in the UK and certain other countries.

Published in the United States of America by Oxford University Press
198 Madison Avenue, New York, NY 10016, United States of America.

© Oxford University Press 2021

Library of Congress Cataloging-in-Publication Data
Names: Han, Paul K. J., author.
Title: Uncertainty in medicine : a framework for tolerance / Paul K.J. Han.
Description: New York, NY : Oxford University Press, [2021] |
Includes bibliographical references and index. |
Identifiers: LCCN 2021004841 (print) | LCCN 2021004842 (ebook) |
ISBN 9780190270582 (paperback) | ISBN 9780190270605 (epub) | ISBN 9780190270612
Subjects: MESH: Philosophy, Medical | Uncertainty | Delivery of Health Care
Classification: LCC R723 (print) | LCC R723 (ebook) | NLM W 61 | DDC 610.1—dc23
LC record available at https://lccn.loc.gov/2021004841
LC ebook record available at https://lccn.loc.gov/2021004842

DOI: 10.1093/oso/9780190270582.001.0001

1 3 5 7 9 8 6 4 2

Printed by Marquis, Canada

The opinions expressed by the author are his own and this material should not be interpreted
as representing the official viewpoint of the U.S. Department of Health and Human Services,
the National Institutes of Health, or the National Cancer Institute.

CONTENTS

CONTENTS

PREFACE

It is with great uncertainty that I put forth this book on uncertainty in medicine. The problem itself is enormous in scope and complexity. Uncertainty pervades every medical experience, arises from numerous sources, focuses on myriad issues, and elicits a wide range of negative and positive psychological responses, ranging from doubt and fear to faith and hope. Because medical problems affect all aspects of human life, medical uncertainties are also tightly interwoven with numerous nonmedical uncertainties about practical and personal matters. The all-encompassing, multifaceted nature of uncertainty makes it impossible to fully capture and tie up in any single, neat package.

At the same time, uncertainty has already been the subject of a large body of scholarly research. Beginning with the late Renée Fox, whose pioneering work in the 1950s established medical uncertainty as a focus of scientific inquiry, leading researchers and clinicians from various disciplines have investigated the phenomenon. Outside of medicine, some of the greatest thinkers throughout history have examined uncertainty as a more general human experience and from a broader range of perspectives, including not only the social sciences but also philosophy, religion, literature, and the arts. Given all that has been previously thought and written about uncertainty—and by minds far greater than my own—I cannot help being acutely aware of my own ignorance about the topic. I know I am simply joining a much larger effort midstream and cannot possibly cover all of the water.

I therefore offer this book with humility, fully acknowledging its many limitations. It is neither a comprehensive account of the entire phenomenon of uncertainty in medicine nor an authoritative synthesis of all relevant empirical evidence and theoretical insights on the topic. It is a personal attempt to better define the phenomenon—to be clearer about what medical uncertainty is, how it affects us, and what is involved in managing it. The book's more modest goal is to provide clinicians and patients with a way of approaching medical uncertainty, an orienting framework that can help them evaluate their own uncertainty and achieve an optimal, adaptive balance in their responses to it. This balance, I believe, is the essence of what it means to tolerate uncertainty and an important but often neglected goal in medicine. To the ultimate question of how to achieve this goal, the book offers no definitive answers—only a way of searching for them. My hope is that the book can at least assist in this search, and hope in this possibility has given me the courage to put it forward.

In this sense, the book itself is an embodiment of uncertainty tolerance. Writing it has required me to balance my own doubt and fear, generated by my personal uncertainty about the value of the effort, with faith and hope. It has made me learn to see my own lack of knowledge as not only a constraining but also a liberating condition that opens up new possibilities. Readers will need a similar capacity to tolerate the many uncertainties that this book leaves unresolved.

Chapter 1

Introduction

The Challenge of Uncertainty in Medicine

What a physician can do to help a patient, then, is often limited. What he ought to do is frequently not clear. And the consequences of his clinical actions cannot always be accurately predicted. Yet, in the face of these uncertainties and limitations, the physician is expected to institute measures which will facilitate the diagnosis and treatment of the problems the patient presents. . . The special difficulty of the physician—the problem that distinguishes him from most other scientists, be they in the fields of pure or applied science—is that the material on which he works is the disease-stricken human being. Thus, the decisions the physician makes, the procedures he carries out, the drugs he prescribes have a proximate, visible, flesh-and-blood impact on the patients under his care. To a significant extent, whether patients get better, get worse, or whether their conditions remain stubbornly fixed is contingent upon what the physician is or is not able to do for them. Because the welfare of the patient is thus directly associated with his actions, the human consequences of his uncertainty, limitation, and fallibility are more apparent to the physician than to most other scientists.

—Renée Fox[1]

As I write these words, our world is engulfed in medical uncertainty. A novel health threat has emerged out of nowhere and turned entire lives upside down. Millions of people have been directly affected by

Uncertainty in Medicine. Paul K.J. Han, Oxford University Press. © Oxford University Press 2021.
DOI: 10.1093/oso/9780190270582.003.0001

this threat, thousands have died from it, and many more have become consumed by dread and fear—locked down and sheltered in place, paralyzed over what to do next.

The health threat responsible for this unprecedented crisis, coronavirus disease 2019 (COVID-19), is teaching us many hard lessons. It is showing how extraordinarily difficult it is to control a pandemic in an interconnected world. It is demonstrating that this task involves more than containing and mitigating a highly contagious pathogen with virulent effects on our physical well-being. It involves containing and mitigating human uncertainty, which is just as contagious and virulent in its effects on our psychological, social, economic, and existential well-being. The COVID-19 pandemic is revealing how uncertainty about a medical problem can cause as much human suffering as the problem itself.

At the same time, the COVID-19 pandemic is also throwing into sharp relief how ill-prepared we are—as individuals, organizations, and societies—to manage medical uncertainty. Our primary management strategy for all health crises is to acquire greater knowledge of the threat at hand. But what strategies should we employ in the meantime? While we wait to cure our ignorance, how should we palliate our uncertainty? Unfortunately, we have no good answers to these questions. As a result, individuals, organizations, and societies are adopting divergent strategies for managing uncertainty about the COVID-19 pandemic, some of which are clearly maladaptive (e.g., forgoing precautionary behaviors, disregarding scientific evidence, perpetuating disinformation, stigmatizing individuals and social groups).

Yet in these respects the COVID-19 pandemic—its massive scale and virulent nature notwithstanding—poses no new challenges; rather, it simply exposes a fundamental problem that has long plagued medicine. Medical uncertainty has always turned entire lives upside down, and its reach extends well beyond any pandemic. Every single day, uncertainty about some other health threat or medical problem is causing someone, somewhere, to be consumed by dread and fear, paralyzed over what to do next, locked down and sheltered in place. For countless patients and clinicians, medical uncertainty is bringing life to a standstill and putting future plans on hold. In this sense the COVID-19 pandemic is simply casting a harsh light on a much broader and long-standing problem and raising the need to better understand and manage it.

Several other contemporary developments and trends in medicine are also raising this need. Ongoing scientific and technological advances, culminating most recently in the sequencing and editing of the human genome, are producing an ever-increasing supply of new medical interventions of promising but unknown value. The evidence-based medicine movement is continuing to generate knowledge of not only the benefits and harms of medical interventions, but the many gaps in this knowledge. A growing emphasis on patient engagement and shared decision making in healthcare is heightening both clinicians' and patients' awareness of these knowledge gaps. Meanwhile, expanding media coverage of scientific controversies about numerous medical interventions—ranging from immunizations to disease screening tests to life-sustaining treatments at the end of life—is extending this awareness to the general public. Together, these and other trends are increasing the production of medical uncertainty, while also exposing our collective ignorance about how to manage it. In spite of the tremendous growth in the volume, visibility, and importance of medical uncertainty in human life, we lack a coherent, systematic, evidence-based approach to managing this uncertainty.

Our collective ignorance about the management of medical uncertainty has multiple causes. Principal among them is what physician and ethicist Jay Katz called a "disregard of uncertainty"—a systemic denial of the existence of uncertainty in medicine, and a collective failure to cope with it.[2] Katz traced this disregard of uncertainty to several sources: the desire to make sense of the world; pressures of "conformity and orthodoxy" in medical practice; specialization in medicine; professional norms and beliefs regarding physicians' responsibility to disclose uncertainty and the consequences of doing so.[2,3] But our collective disregard of medical uncertainty, I believe, stems from even more fundamental sources. One is a basic human impulse that the great psychologist, philosopher, and physician William James—whose seminal ideas I reference extensively throughout this book—called the "hope of truth": the "faith that truth exists, and that our minds can find it."[4] In medicine, this hope of truth drives every clinical and scientific endeavor, every act of caring and discovery. Yet this same hope also prevents us from treating uncertainty as anything but an intellectual deficit to be corrected by greater knowledge.

Compounding our collective disregard of medical uncertainty and our resulting ignorance about its management is the pervasiveness of uncertainty as a more general aspect of our lives. Uncertainty is an inseparable part of all human endeavors; every activity of daily living—every question we ask, every rule we follow, every decision we make—is a response to our ignorance about some aspect of the world. Our ignorance, furthermore, is so integral to our everyday lives that we ignore our subjective experience of it. We focus our attention outward on the things we do not know, rather than inward on our state of not knowing: we devote our effort to eliminating our ignorance rather than managing our uncertainty. Like the air we breathe, uncertainty becomes invisible to us, and the same is true in medicine. The things we do not know about any given medical problem are so numerous and consequential that they command all of our attention and consume all of our energy as clinicians and patients. Every single activity of clinical care—every medical history and physical examination performed, every diagnostic test ordered, every medical and surgical treatment rendered—focuses on closing objective gaps in our medical knowledge, as opposed to coping with our subjective experience of these gaps. Medical uncertainty is so pervasive, in other words, that we simply take it for granted and devote little conscious effort to understanding and managing it.

Another important cause of our ignorance about the management of medical uncertainty is its complex, fundamentally ambiguous nature. Medical uncertainty comes in a wide variety of sizes, shapes, and forms. It arises from various sources and pertains to numerous issues, both scientific and nonscientific. It produces a variety of psychological responses, both negative and positive, that vary depending on what it represents for different individuals in different situations. On the one hand, uncertainty represents the possibility of a bad outcome and is thus a negative experience. It provokes fear for the 70-year-old grandfather, retired schoolteacher and nursing home resident, living in the midst of a COVID-19 outbreak in his facility. For the exhausted front-line healthcare workers at this facility, uncertainty elicits numerous other negative responses, including anger, resentment, and burnout. On the other hand, uncertainty represents the possibility of a good outcome and is thus a positive experience. It offers hope for the 40-year-old emergency room nurse suffering from severe COVID-19 pneumonia, hospitalized in the intensive care unit of her own hospital, and receiving an unproven new therapeutic agent through a clinical trial. For physicians like the one caring for this patient, furthermore, uncertainty elicits other positive responses, including curiosity and professional satisfaction; it is "the very muse that inspires the intellectual fascination of medical practice," as surgeon and writer Sherwin Nuland put it.[5] Uncertainty in medicine is thus both an affliction and a fundamental human need: We can't live with it, but we can't live without it. The dual, paradoxical nature of uncertainty further compounds the difficulty of understanding and managing it.

A final important cause of our collective ignorance about the management of medical uncertainty is its inseparability from other more fundamental, nonmedical uncertainties. These include epistemological uncertainties regarding the nature and limits of human knowledge; moral uncertainties regarding the appropriate standards of human behavior; and existential uncertainties regarding the ultimate meaning and purpose of human life. These uncertainties normally lie latent and unaddressed, but become manifest during times of crisis—as the COVID-19 pandemic is currently demonstrating. Clinical interventions for this novel health threat—ranging from hydroxychloroquine and remdesivir, to monoclonal antibody therapy, to vaccines still under development—raise epistemological questions about the nature and extent of scientific knowledge and the standards of evidence used to justify medical interventions. Public health interventions—ranging from mandated lockdowns and travel bans to recommended behaviors such as mask wearing—raise moral questions about the acceptability of competing risks, the appropriateness of limits to personal freedom, and the relative value of health compared to other human goods. Finally, COVID-19 itself raises existential questions—what sociologist Renée Fox called "metaquestions" pertaining to "the 'whys' of pain, suffering, the limits of human life, and death, and about their relations to evil, sin, and injustice"—that demand more than scientific answers.[6] The inseparability of medical uncertainty from all of these fundamental nonmedical uncertainties further constrains our collective ability to understand and manage it.

MEETING THE CHALLENGE: A FRAMEWORK FOR TOLERANCE

Although medical uncertainty is an extremely important problem to understand and manage, its pervasiveness, complexity, and ambiguity lead us to disregard it. We focus our attention on the objective gaps in our knowledge rather than our subjective experience of these gaps—that is, on ignorance rather than uncertainty. This systemic disregard has important self-reinforcing consequences. It leads us to treat medical uncertainty as a pathological condition to be eradicated through the pursuit of knowledge, rather than a normal state of being to be accepted and managed through other means. It focuses our efforts on curing uncertainty, rather than palliating its effects. Medical uncertainty consequently becomes even more overwhelming, which fuels even greater efforts to eradicate it. Because perfect knowledge in medicine is unattainable, however, these efforts ultimately lead to disappointment and frustration and leave the underlying problem unaddressed.

This situation is no longer tenable. If for no other reason than the COVID-19 pandemic, the need to understand and manage medical uncertainty has reached a tipping point. The widespread human suffering caused by medical uncertainty compels us to break the vicious cycle of our systemic disregard of medical uncertainty and our collective ignorance about its management. It calls on us to expand the paradigm of medicine to include not only the cure but also the palliation of medical uncertainty—to devote equal attention to helping clinicians and patients live with it.

This book offers a potential starting point for this effort: a conceptual framework that can enable clinicians and patients to approach the problem of medical uncertainty in an organized manner. To develop this framework, the book examines the nature, causes, and effects of uncertainty as a more general human experience. It synthesizes insights from disciplines beyond medicine—the social sciences and philosophy in particular—to develop a descriptive framework of the variety of uncertainties that arise in medicine and the diverse, often conflicting ways that people respond to them. It goes on to propose a working definition of uncertainty tolerance and a normative framework to guide efforts to increase this tolerance. The book's working hypothesis is that an organizing framework can enable clinicians and patients to tolerate uncertainty by transcending it: achieving a higher-order metacognitive perspective that allows them to regulate their own responses to uncertainty.

I put forth this conceptual framework recognizing the many challenges and limitations of the effort. The vast scope of existing literature on uncertainty, both in and outside medicine, makes a truly comprehensive synthesis impossible. The framework is thus necessarily incomplete and provisional. Empirical evidence on the causes, effects, and management of uncertainty is limited and evolving. The framework is thus necessarily speculative—based as much on my own perspectives, values, and experiences as a clinician, researcher, and human being as on established scientific knowledge. Finally, conceptual frameworks are merely mental models that impose a logical form, structure, and order on reality. The current framework is thus necessarily abstract—composed of idealized constructs that can never fully capture the richness and complexity of medical uncertainty as a lived experience.

Yet these limitations, I believe, do not undermine the value of this framework. In the final analysis, a conceptual framework need not provide a perfect, complete representation of a given phenomenon. It simply needs to be useful to some purpose, and that is the goal of the framework presented in this book. It is neither an exhaustive phenomenological description nor a grand causal theory of medical uncertainty. It is a basic road map—a navigational tool designed to help clinicians and patients evaluate and manage their uncertainties.

In developing this framework, I adopt the heuristic strategy of treating medical uncertainty as a health problem—a type of "illness"—and describe it using the same conceptual categories that medical textbooks use to characterize all health problems: nature, etiology, anatomy, natural history, and management. Similarly, I describe the management of uncertainty in terms of the prototypical clinical tasks familiar to physicians and other health professionals: making a diagnosis, assessing prognosis, determining appropriate treatment. Of course, this analogy cannot be pushed too far; uncertainty is not a pathological condition, but a normal, inescapable part of human life. As I hope to show, however, the established conceptual categories and clinical tasks of medicine provide a useful way of approaching not only health problems but also our uncertainty about them and a coherent scaffolding for an organizing framework.

The framework has several parts, which correspond to different aspects of medical uncertainty that I analyze in turn. I begin in Chapter 2 by examining the nature of uncertainty and introducing a working definition of the phenomenon as a metacognitive awareness of ignorance. I show how this metacognitive awareness is both psychologically generated by novelty, discrepancy, and deliberation, and socially constructed and transmitted. In Chapter 3, I describe the anatomy of uncertainty in terms of its fundamental sources (root causes), issues (substantive problems), and loci (persons in whose minds uncertainty resides) and develop a conceptual framework that classifies the variety of uncertainties in medicine according to these three dimensions. In Chapter 4, I describe the natural history of uncertainty—that is, the way that uncertainty manifests in people's lives—in terms of two types of responses to uncertainty: primary (initial cognitive, emotional, and behavioral responses) and secondary (compensatory responses aimed at regulating primary responses). I develop a conceptual framework that classifies the variety of both primary and secondary responses to uncertainty. In Chapter 5, I shift from a descriptive to a normative mode of analysis and explore the terra incognita of how to manage medical uncertainty. I discuss the concept of "uncertainty tolerance" as an aspirational goal that supplements—rather than supplants—medicine's principal goal of acquiring knowledge and reducing uncertainty. I introduce a working definition of uncertainty tolerance as the capacity to achieve an optimal, adaptive balance in our diverse responses to uncertainty and argue that this capacity encompasses three key moral virtues: humility, flexibility, and courage. I present an integrative practical framework of uncertainty management that identifies four key tasks in the effort: establishing the diagnosis of uncertainty, assessing its prognosis, clarifying goals, and initiating treatment. In Chapter 6, I conclude the book by offering a vision for how to promote uncertainty tolerance in medicine. I identify various system-level strategies—spanning medical care, education, and research—that can foster humility, flexibility, and courage and thereby help build uncertainty tolerance into the structures and processes of healthcare. I argue that these strategies ultimately enable uncertainty tolerance to become part of both the worldview of individual clinicians and patients and the overall culture of medicine.

In the end, a conceptual framework alone cannot change reality, but it can help us adapt to it. The framework put forth in this book offers no final, universal answers to the question of how individual clinicians or patients should manage the particular uncertainties they experience—only a particular approach to searching for answers. It also provides no way of eliminating the suffering caused by medical uncertainty—only a particular orientation toward this suffering. Whether the framework will ultimately prove useful in spite of these limitations remains to be seen. My hope, however, is that it can be a momentary source of help to clinicians, patients, and others who are struggling with the unknowns of medicine: a stepping stone in an ongoing journey toward uncertainty tolerance.

Note: In the epigraph and several quotations in this book, the original authors use the words *man, men,* or masculine pronouns to refer to clinicians, people, or humankind in general. Such usage is currently not socially acceptable; however, this was not the case at the time of the original writings, and for the sake of fidelity to these writings I have left them unaltered.

Chapter 2

The Nature and Etiology
of Uncertainty

So long as an object is unusual, our expectations are baffled; they are
fully determined as soon as it becomes familiar.... Everyone knows how
when a painful thing has to be undergone in the near future, the vague
feeling that it is impending penetrates all our thought with uneasiness
and subtly vitiates our mood even when it does not control our atten-
tion; it keeps us from being at rest, at home in the given present. The
same is true when a great happiness awaits us. But when the future is
neutral and perfectly certain, "we do not mind it," as we say, but give an
undisturbed attention to the actual. Let now this haunting sense of futu-
rity be thrown off its bearings or left without an object, and immediately
uneasiness takes possession of the mind. But in every novel or unclassified
experience this is just what occurs; we do not know what will come next,
and novelty per se becomes a mental irritant, while custom per se is a
mental sedative, merely because the one baffles while the other settles our
expectations.

—William James[1]

The first task in developing a conceptual framework of medical uncertainty is to establish a coherent understanding of the nature and etiology of uncertainty as a more general phenomenon. The challenge,
however, is that uncertainty has been understood in many different
ways that need to be reconciled. To this end, I begin my analysis by

Uncertainty in Medicine. Paul K.J. Han, Oxford University Press. © Oxford University Press 2021.
DOI: 10.1093/oso/9780190270582.003.0002

exploring these different understandings and proposing a working definition of uncertainty as a metacognitive state that is both psychologically and socially constructed and transmitted.

THE MANY MEANINGS OF UNCERTAINTY

Dictionary definitions of uncertainty capture several different meanings of the term. The *Merriam-Webster Dictionary*, for example, defines uncertainty as "the state of being uncertain" and uses a plethora of terms to define uncertain: indefinite, indeterminate, not certain to occur, problematical, not reliable, untrustworthy, not known beyond doubt, dubious, doubtful, not clearly identified or defined, not constant, variable, and fitful.[2] The *Oxford English Dictionary* defines uncertainty using a similarly broad range of terms that signify four different types of phenomena: (1) a *state of mind* (the "state or character of being uncertain in mind," or the "quality or state of being uncertain"); (2) a *state of being* (the "state of not being definitely known or perfectly clear"); (3) an *object* ("something of which the occurrence, results, etc., is uncertain" or "something not definitely known or knowable"); and (4) a *feature of an object* (the "quality of being uncertain," a "liability to chance or accident," the "quality of being indeterminate," or an "amount of variation").[3]

These alternative definitions are incompatible; strictly speaking, uncertainty cannot simultaneously be a state of mind, a state of being, an object, and a feature of an object. Furthermore, definitions of uncertainty as an object or feature are tautological; they depend on a prior designation of a given object or feature as "uncertain" or "not definitely known or knowable," by a conscious subject who is able to first experience uncertainty as a state of mind or being. In other words, it is not the object or feature of the object that is uncertain; it is the human being who perceives and designates it as such. Uncertainty is ultimately a subjective rather than an objective phenomenon, a mental state rather than a material "thing" residing in the extra-mental world. It lies entirely in the eye and mind of the beholder.

Uncertainty as a metacognition

But if uncertainty represents a subjective mental state, what specifically defines this state? Lack of knowledge is the quintessential characteristic highlighted in dictionary definitions; however, uncertainty signifies more than ignorance alone. Subjective definitions of uncertainty use several descriptors (e.g., indefiniteness, dubious, doubtfulness) that imply not only ignorance about some aspect of reality but also a higher-order, self-reflective awareness of this ignorance, which is necessary for one to be indefinite, dubious, or doubtful in the first place.

In other words, uncertainty is a metacognition—one of several self-reflective mental states consisting of "knowledge concerning one's own cognitive processes and products or anything related to them," as psychologist John Flavell originally defined it.[4] Metacognition explains "how one and the same organ can be the organ doing the observing and the organ being observed,"[5] and represents a higher, second-order, metalevel cognitive process directed at the mind's lower, primary-level cognitions, which are directed at objects of the external world.

Uncertainty is a specific type of metacognition consisting of the subjective perception of one's ignorance—that is, one's lower-level lack of knowledge—about some aspect of the world.[6,7] It is this metacognitive perception that is captured by conventional definitions of uncertainty, for example feelings of doubt, perceptions of indefiniteness, indeterminacy, unreliability, and so on. The psychological opposite of uncertainty is the metacognition of certainty—the subjective mental experience of having knowledge[5,8]—which William James long ago described as a feeling of knowing:

> *Of some things we feel that we are certain: we know, and we know that we do know. There is something that gives a click inside of us, a bell that strikes twelve, when the hands of our mental clock have swept the dial and meet over the meridian hour.*[9]

Uncertainty, however, is not the absence of the feeling of knowing, but a feeling of the absence of knowing: the subjective perception of the lack of knowledge.

In this metacognitive conception, the existence of uncertainty is jointly determined by two principal factors: (1) absence of understanding and (2) presence of conscious awareness. Figure 2.1 illustrates how both factors are necessary; either gaining

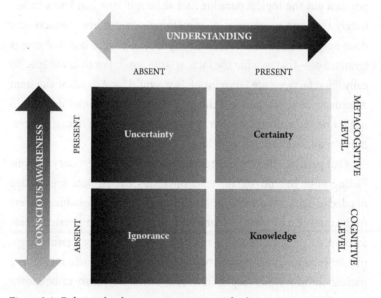

Figure 2.1 Relationship between uncertainty and other epistemic states.

understanding or losing one's awareness of ignorance would move one to a different epistemic state (certainty, ignorance, knowledge). In medicine, both patients and clinicians continuously move in and out of uncertainty in these ways. The 40-year-old emergency room nurse and mother of two with a three-day history of a dry cough and a fever resides in an initial, vague state of ignorance about her health; she does not know whether she even has a health problem, let alone what the specific problem might be. At some point, however, her suffering drives her to raise these questions, and she moves from ignorance to uncertainty about her health—from a state of simply not knowing to a state of knowing that there is something she does not know.

The metacognitive knowledge embodied by uncertainty, however, is necessarily imprecise: It does not include exactly *what* one does not know, for this would require the very knowledge that ignorance, by definition, precludes. Philosopher Nicholas Rescher pointed out the logical paradox that although "one can know indefinitely that one is ignorant of something—that there are facts one does not know—one cannot know specifically what it is that one is ignorant of—that is, what the facts at issue are."[10] For to know specifically what facts we are ignorant of, "we would have to know the item at issue to be a fact, and just this is, by hypothesis, something we do not know."[11] Achieving greater specificity or precision in one's uncertainty requires more information.

Our patient achieves greater precision in her uncertainty by consulting with her physician, who possesses the clinical knowledge needed to generate a differential diagnosis—a list of possible answers to the question of what is wrong with the patient. The physician performs a set of clinical tasks—taking a medical history, performing a physical examination, conducting diagnostic tests—and educates the patient about various diagnostic possibilities previously unbeknown to the patient. At this point her uncertainty becomes more specific; she comes to know more precisely what she does not know.

The diagnostic workup eventually produces an unfortunate answer: SARS-CoV-2 (severe acute respiratory syndrome coronavirus 2) infection. With this new knowledge, both the patient and the physician achieve diagnostic certainty, that is, the feeling of knowing what the health problem is. But they do not exit the state of uncertainty, for they then become aware of many other things they do not know: what treatment options are best for this patient; what side effects she will suffer; how her illness and treatment will affect her family and loved ones; whether and how long she will survive her illness. Medical uncertainty remains; its focus simply shifts to other issues of ignorance. Only with the passage of time, as medical reality declares itself, do the patient and the physician move from ignorance to knowledge, uncertainty to certainty.

The epistemic states of uncertainty, certainty, ignorance, and knowledge, however, are not completely discrete and categorical in nature. The boundaries separating them are not definite or fixed because both knowledge and awareness are also not categorical but continuous phenomena that vary in degree. The blurred borders in Figure 2.1 are meant to convey the indefinite nature of the boundaries separating uncertainty and other epistemic states. These boundaries, furthermore, are not static but constantly shifting. William James famously described human consciousness as a dynamic phenomenon—an ever-flowing "stream" of multiple "sensibly continuous" states in constant flux.[12] As specific forms of consciousness, uncertainty, certainty, ignorance, and knowledge are also processes in dynamic equilibrium—shifting currents within the broader stream of consciousness, which are defined by their relationship to one another. Compared to these other currents, uncertainty may be weaker or stronger, more or less latent or manifest at any given moment. At no time, however, does it disappear completely; it merely submerges and resurfaces in our awareness at different times.

As subjective metacognitions, uncertainty and certainty also vary in their respective relationships with ignorance and knowledge; there is no simple 1:1 correlation between them. Individuals can experience uncertainty despite being knowledgeable or, conversely, certainty despite being ignorant. During the COVID-19 pandemic, for example, some individuals have chosen not to wear face coverings to prevent transmission of the SARS-CoV-2 virus; this choice is due to a conviction that they are not at personal risk of either contracting or transmitting the infection or that masks are ineffective. In other words, individuals can experience "false" uncertainty or certainty—that is, a relative level of uncertainty or certainty that is disproportionate to a given level of ignorance or knowledge. However, the appropriate level of uncertainty or certainty for any given individual or situation is a complex moral judgment that depends on various factors, including personal values, needs, and dispositions, as well as situational demands for certainty versus uncertainty. Personality differences, for example, may predispose some patients and clinicians to feel more certain than others at a given level of personal knowledge. Similarly, serious medical conditions demanding urgent intervention (e.g., severe COVID-19 pneumonia with rapid clinical deterioration, acute myocardial infarction requiring emergent revascularization) may predispose patients and clinicians to feel more certain than they normally would with the same level of knowledge, given the pressing need to take action.

THE METACOGNITIVE FUNCTIONS OF UNCERTAINTY

As a metacognitive state, uncertainty is justified by the fundamental limitations to all human knowledge. It represents the intellectually honest acknowledgment of these limitations, which great thinkers since antiquity have lauded as a moral ideal. Confucius regarded true wisdom as the capacity "to know what you know and know what you do not know,"[13] and Plato is thought to have ascribed this same capacity to Socrates.[14] Yet uncertainty is not only morally justified by the fundamental limitations of all human knowledge, but psychologically justified by the adaptive regulatory functions it serves.

Flavell argued that metacognition serves the primary function of allowing individuals to both monitor and control their cognitive activities.[4] Metacognition consists of an individual's knowledge about their own cognitive abilities, the strategies and tasks they must employ to think and take action, and the expected outcomes of different courses of action. It also consists of metacognitive experiences—individuals' "conscious cognitive or affective experiences that accompany and pertain to any intellectual enterprise."[4] Metacognitive knowledge and experiences not only enable individuals to monitor their own thoughts and cognitive activities, but also to control them: to "select, evaluate, revise, and abandon cognitive tasks, goals, and strategies in light of their relationships with one another" and individuals' own abilities and interests.[5] Whereas monitoring is a "bottom-up" process through which cognitions are represented to the knowing self, control is a "top-down" process through which the knowing self manages cognitions in order to adapt to the world and achieve one's goals.[5,15,16]

Metacognition thus serves a broader introspective "executive function" of cognitive *regulation*.[4] In contrast to lower-level cognitions, which constitute representations of objects in the extra-mental world, metacognitions constitute higher-level representations of one's own mental representations and of how they apply to the extra-mental world.[17] These higher-level representations enable individuals to understand, plan, predict, and assess their own reactions to problems they confront and thereby respond more effectively. There is no theoretical limit, furthermore, to the number of levels of metacognitions; mental representations can themselves become the object of cognitions and representations at still higher levels.

Researchers have also identified several types of metacognitions, including judgments of learning, ease of learning, familiarity, confidence, and task difficulty, which serve a variety of adaptive, regulatory functions.[16,18,19] For example, judgments of task difficulty induce negative affect and initiation of deliberation, information seeking, and other goal-oriented actions, while judgments of familiarity induce positive affect and cessation of deliberation and information seeking. As a broader metacognition, uncertainty also serves adaptive regulatory functions. It enables individuals to recognize their ignorance and take appropriate action (e.g., withholding judgment, seeking more information, delaying or exercising caution, restraint, and prudence in decision-making). It prevents the metaignorant unawareness of one's own knowledge deficits and the consequent overestimation of one's cognitive abilities—a common cognitive bias that psychologist David Dunning characterized as the "anosognosia of everyday life,"[20] in reference to the pathological lack of self-awareness exhibited by patients with stroke, traumatic brain injury, and dementia. A large body of empirical research has led this lack of awareness to be known as the Dunning-Kruger effect.[21,22] Leonid Rozenblit and Frank Keil have described it as an overconfidence bias, an "illusion of explanatory depth" consisting of a powerful but inaccurate sense of knowledge that arises when "people feel they understand complex phenomena with far greater precision, coherence, and depth than they really do."[23] Steven Sloman has described this bias more broadly as a "knowledge illusion."[24]

Uncertainty is an antidote against these powerful cognitive biases. It is an essential form of knowledge that serves the broader metacognitive function of increasing our awareness of our ignorance, thereby enabling us to think and act more wisely. Uncertainty prompts the young woman with a cough and fever to stop and think about the possibility of an illness such as COVID-19, rather than simply dismissing her symptoms as ordinary and benign. Uncertainty protects the patient's primary care physician from overconfidence in her own clinical judgment and physical examination skills and from simply assuming that her initial diagnosis is correct. It makes her pause to think twice before simply acting; to consider the broadest possible range of diagnostic possibilities; to reconsider her initial diagnostic or therapeutic plan; and to seek a second opinion from a colleague. It represents not only a mental state but also an attitude that Sextus Empiricus and the ancient Skeptic philosophers described as a "suspension of judgment"[25,26]—an active noncommitment to any particular belief about the world. Philosopher Jane Friedman further characterized this attitude as a "committed neutrality"—a dedication to "keeping lines of inquiry open but 'paused' "[27] rather than settling and answering the questions at hand.[28] Friedman observed that our ignorance occupies "a vast space of possibilities" and normally goes unnoticed. When we suspend judgment, however, "we frame up some portion of this space of the unknown. . . . We move ourselves from a state of mere ignorance, to explicit uncertainty: we bring some aspect of the unknown into view."[27] Uncertainty is the attitude of committed neutrality that opens our eyes to our ignorance.

Of course, the doubt-promoting metacognitive function of uncertainty is not always adaptive. Human cognitive resources are finite, and the demands of everyday life make it impossible to devote continuous, undivided attention to all we do not know. Excessive uncertainty, furthermore, can interfere with our ability to act; it can promote an endless search for information and either a corresponding delay or a complete avoidance of decision-making. Rozenblit and Keil have thus argued that "it may therefore be quite adaptive to have the illusion that we know more than we do so that we settle for what is enough," rather than engaging in "potentially inexhaustible searches for ever-deeper understanding."[23] At some point we need to suppress our uncertainty and cease our efforts to reduce it and simply move ahead with our lives. At some point we need to engage in an even higher-level, metacognitive regulatory process focused on managing uncertainty itself.

THE ETIOLOGY OF UNCERTAINTY: PSYCHOLOGICAL ORIGINS

Having established a working definition of uncertainty as the metacognitive, subjective perception or state of awareness of ignorance, the next task is to establish its etiology. What prompts individuals to achieve this higher-order, self-reflective awareness? William James long ago contended that it is the unusual, "novel or unclassified" nature of a given experience, which baffles expectations and "keeps us from being at rest, at home in the given present."[1] More recently, developmental psychologist Jerome Kagan similarly attributed uncertainty to the novelty or discrepancy of an experience with respect to existing mental representations.[29] Building on the work of Piaget, Kagan argued that these mental representations consist of two main types: schemata and semantic networks. Schemata are more primitive, visceral or perceptual representations that are used primarily for recognition of events and objects experienced in the past, and form the basis of unconscious knowledge. Semantic networks, on the other hand, are more advanced conceptual representations that are used for classification, reason, inference, and communication, and form the basis of conscious knowledge.

Kagan argued that novelty and discrepancy produce two distinct phenomenological states, depending on the type of mental representation involved: (1) surprise, as a lower-order, subconscious, brief, immediate, and automatic state produced by the perceptual novelty and discrepancy of an experience compared to lower-order schematic representations; and (2) uncertainty, as a higher-order, conscious, prolonged, deliberative cognitive state provoked by the conceptual novelty or discrepancy of an experience compared to existing semantic representations.[29] In the domain of medicine, examples of stimuli that engender surprise include unfamiliar or inconsistent symptoms, while stimuli that engender uncertainty include unfamiliar interpretations of these symptoms or conflicting information about an individual's diagnosis, prognosis, or treatment.

What Kagan's conception makes clear is that although novelty and discrepancy are necessary for uncertainty, they are not sufficient; active deliberation is also necessary. For novelty or discrepancy about any aspect of reality to give rise to uncertainty, they must be more than simply *perceived* at an elemental, subconscious level. They must be *conceived* at a higher-order, conscious level; they must become objects of conscious thought. Uncertainty, in other words, entails a fundamental shift from an automatic to a deliberative mode of cognition. "Dual-process" theories of human thinking and reasoning, put forth by psychologists Keith Stanovich, Richard West, and others, provide a useful way of thinking about this cognitive shift. These theories posit two main modes of thinking: System 1 and System 2.[30–32] System 1 thinking is automatic, unconscious, implicit, concrete, intuitive, and heuristic-based,[32,33] and operates automatically and rapidly, with little or no effort or sense of voluntary control.[33] System 2 thinking, in contrast, is deliberate, conscious, explicit, abstract, logical, and analytical, and operates intentionally and slowly, consuming significant cognitive resources.[32]

Each mode of thinking serves different psychological functions. Daniel Kahneman argued that System 1 thinking provides a continuous assessment of the problems that an organism must solve to survive.[33] System 1 thinking does not solve these problems actively and deliberatively, but passively and expediently; it "suppresses ambiguity and spontaneously constructs stories that are as coherent as possible," leading people to "jump to conclusions."[33] It operates at the lower cognitive level of "surprise" in Kagan's conception. System 2 thinking, in contrast, focuses on active, deliberative problem-solving. As Kahneman put it, System 2 thinking takes over when things get difficult—whenever "a question arises for which System 1 does not offer an answer" (p. 86). It operates exclusively at the higher cognitive level of "uncertainty" in Kagan's conception. Kahneman underscored the dependence of uncertainty on deliberative, System 2 thinking: "Conscious doubt is not in the repertoire of System 1; it requires maintaining incompatible interpretations in mind at the same time, which demands mental effort. Uncertainty and doubt are the domain of System 2."[34]

Uncertainty thus ultimately depends on the joint occurrence of two psychological conditions: (1) novelty or discrepancy in an event or proposition and (2) active deliberation. Each condition gives rise to a different essential component of uncertainty; novelty and discrepancy give rise to ignorance, while active deliberation gives rise to the metacognitive awareness of this ignorance. To experience uncertainty, in other words, the primary care physician evaluating the patient with an unexplained pneumonia must not only lack knowledge of the diagnosis, but also actively reflect on her lack of knowledge. Through this quantum leap of deliberation she changes her relationship to her ignorance in a fundamental way: She rises above it.

THE ETIOLOGY OF UNCERTAINTY: SOCIAL ORIGINS

But the etiology of uncertainty is not exclusively psychological, given that the mental representations—what Kagan called semantic networks—that determine the relative novelty or discrepancy of life experiences and the uncertainty they generate do not simply arise ex nihilo from an individual's solitary intrapsychic experiences. Rather, these representations are inherited from a preexisting cultural repository of knowledge that originates beyond the individual. The etiology of uncertainty, therefore, lies not only in the psychological processes that give rise to the metacognitive awareness of ignorance, but also in the social processes that give rise to the mental representations that shape this awareness.

Medical anthropologist and psychiatrist Arthur Kleinman put forth a useful approach to understanding these representations and the social processes that give rise to them in his influential concept of explanatory models (EMs): "notions about an episode of sickness and its treatment that are employed by all those engaged in the clinical process."[35] EMs provide answers to key questions about specific health conditions, including their etiology, symptoms, pathophysiology, natural history, and treatment and come in a range of forms, from logical propositions to numeric probabilities. They embody the collective, cumulative knowledge of different groups of people and vary in authorship and content. Professional EMs authored and adopted by clinicians, for example, focus largely on scientific concerns, while lay EMs authored and adopted by patients are broader in scope.[35]

In the etiology of uncertainty, EMs are the preexisting mental representations that originate from beyond individuals and give rise to uncertainty in two important ways. First, they provide the background knowledge that determines what problems individuals perceive as novel or discrepant and thus how much uncertainty they experience. Early in the COVID-19 pandemic, for example, when an adequate scientific EM for the "pneumonia of unknown cause" was lacking, every aspect of the illness—from its clinical presentation and natural history to its prevention and treatment—was novel and uncertainty provoking. As medical knowledge expanded and a more complete EM emerged, however, the novelty of at least some of these aspects of COVID-19 wore off, and their associated uncertainty correspondingly diminished. Of course, much remains unknown about COVID-19, and individual clinicians' and patients' overall uncertainty about the illness may be not so much diminished as simply redirected toward different unknowns. However, the larger point is that EMs mediate this entire process by establishing the epistemic boundaries between the known and the unknown that, when violated, give rise to uncertainty.

The other important way in which EMs give rise to uncertainty is by allowing the conscious awareness of ignorance to be transmitted from one individual to another. Kleinman viewed EMs as portable goods that individuals exchange through various "transactional processes" (pp. 111–113). These include the elicitation and analysis of an EM, its transfer and restructuring within one's own, and its feedback or influence on EMs of other individuals. These processes can occur in a direct and personal manner (e.g., through clinical encounters between health professionals and patients). They are formalized in the ideal of shared decision-making (SDM), which physician and researcher Glyn Elwyn has construed as a process of "collaborative deliberation" in which health professionals and patients work together to understand how best to manage a particular health problem.[36–41] The concept of SDM signifies a two-way transaction: The clinician provides the patient with scientific information on the expected benefits, harms, and uncertainties of the medical options at hand, while the patient provides the clinician with personal information on his or her values and preferences.[36,38,39] Conceived in terms of Kleinman's model, SDM is a social process in which the professional, scientific EM of the clinician and the personal, lay EM of the patient are exchanged, and new knowledge is co-constructed. Yet the exchange of EMs can also occur in an indirect, impersonal manner, such as through passive exposure to information from news media channels or active search and exchange of information on the Internet and social media. In such situations, the elicitation, transfer, restructuring, and feedback of EMs occur virtually and more anonymously.

Through these transactional processes EMs transmit knowledge and certainty; they are "the main vehicle for the clinical construction of reality," as Kleinman has put it.[35] At the same time, EMs are also the main vector for the person-to-person transmission of ignorance and uncertainty, which can occur either separately or simultaneously. Early in course of the COVID-19 pandemic, for example, the prevailing EM put forth by US government officials recommended against the use of face coverings to prevent spread of the novel coronavirus, based upon the lack of scientific evidence for their effectiveness. Unacknowledged and subsequently lost in the public translation of this EM, however, was the fact that lack of evidence for effectiveness is not equivalent to evidence for the lack of effectiveness, and that the true effectiveness of mask use was unknown. The prevailing EM thus transmitted ignorance without uncertainty: it perpetuated the erroneous view that masks were ineffective, while failing to acknowledge that existing evidence was insufficient to recommend either for or against mask use. The outcome was excessive public certainty about a mistaken belief.

The situation changed when evidence on the effectiveness of masks and the extent of asymptomatic and airborne transmission of the novel coronavirus virus began to emerge. Public health and government officials responded by acknowledging the potential benefits of masks in preventing viral spread and advocating their use. Other officials disagreed, however, and what is now playing out in American society is a conflict between a growing number of divergent EMs— some favoring mask use, others opposing it—that manifest variability in the standards of evidence used to evaluate public health interventions and in the underlying values, concerns, worldviews, and motivations of different groups of people. What these divergent EMs have in common, however, is a focus on maintaining uncertainty. Without a shared, conscious awareness of ignorance about the true effectiveness of masks, there would be no legitimate conflict; the issue would simply be resolved. Both proponents and opponents of mask use thus strive to raise and reinforce this awareness. They transmit EMs that not only advocate for or against mask use, but also highlight the persistence of scientific uncertainty arising from various sources: the limitations of existing evidence, the inherent unpredictability of viral spread, the inability of any expert to determine whether any single individual will benefit from masks or other preventive measures. Uncertainty arising from these and other sources keeps the issue of mask use alive for both proponents and opponents—leaving open the possibility that their own EMs represent the correct course of action.

Explanatory models transmit uncertainty, furthermore, not only by highlighting scientific ignorance but also by conveying information that casts doubt on alternative EMs. This endeavor can be legitimate—as when EMs introduce new evidence or interpretations that conflict with the old. However, it can also be illegitimate—as when EMs put forth conflicting interpretations or draw attention to scientific ignorance solely as a means of "manufacturing doubt," as epidemiologist David Michaels has put it,[42] that serves strategic ends. Such EMs may be the products of intentional disinformation campaigns aimed at distorting or suppressing scientific evidence or disseminating false information that both exaggerates the extent of scientific uncertainty and also weaponizes it. Michaels and others have documented the efforts of the tobacco and oil industries, for example, to put forth EMs that deliberately magnified the extent of scientific uncertainty about the health effects of tobacco and the origins and environmental effects of climate change, respectively, in order to advance their own economic interests. Examples from the current pandemic include the promulgation of alternative

EMs—some of which have been shaped and legitimized by government officials—that leverage scientific uncertainty to dismiss the effectiveness of mask use and other risk-reducing measures, and even deny the very existence of COVID-19.

A full account of the many complex cultural, social, economic, and political factors and processes that give rise to these and other EMs is well beyond the scope of the current analysis. The important point is that these various processes occur both inside and outside of the minds of individuals, and that the production and transmission of uncertainty are thus both psychological and social processes. The concept of EMs helps us think about uncertainty as a communicable condition—constructed, inherited, accepted or rejected, reconstructed, and ultimately passed on from one person to another. EMs are the preexisting, culturally derived, socially constructed mental representations that mediate these processes; uncertainty arises when the EMs residing in the mind of one clinician, patient, or other individual comes into contact with EMs residing in the mind of another.

TOWARD AN EXPLANATORY MODEL OF UNCERTAINTY

I have put forth a conception of uncertainty as a metacognitive state that is psychologically induced by novelty, discrepancy, and deliberation and socially constructed and transmitted through the exchange of EMs. In this conception, uncertainty originates from a deficit of knowledge, but paradoxically represents a higher-level, adaptive form of knowledge—a "learned ignorance which is conscious of itself," as Pascal put it.[43] This learned ignorance serves the essential function of helping us respond appropriately to novelty and discrepancy. It prevents overconfidence, promotes precautionary actions (e.g., withholding judgment, seeking information, deferring decisions), and enables us to be open to new knowledge and experiences.

This conception of uncertainty, of course, is itself an EM built out of a body of preexisting knowledge. Like all EMs, it is a cultural artifact that orders and "reifies" some subjective human experience, as sociologists Peter Berger and Thomas Luckmann put it—transforming it into an objective reality existing outside of us.[44] Like all EMs, it challenges prior knowledge and thus produces both questions and answers, uncertainty and certainty. Unlike most EMs, however, this EM deals specifically with our uncertainty itself—the subjective experience of ignorance that drives the production and transmission of EMs to begin with—as opposed to the concrete objects of our ignorance. It orders and reifies this unique subjective experience, turning it into an object we can stand apart from and act on. It has the practical potential to help us manage our uncertainty.

To realize this potential, however, the EM must first be given additional shape and form. Acting on our uncertainty requires understanding not only its nature and etiology, but also its composition. We need to adequately describe the anatomy of uncertainty—to break it down into its essential elements and to account for its various manifestations in medicine. I now turn to this task.

Chapter 3

The Anatomy of Uncertainty

In the suspense of uncertainty, we metaphorically climb a tree; we try to find some standpoint from which we may survey additional facts and, getting a more commanding view of the situation, may decide how the facts stand related to one another.

—John Dewey[1]

The anatomical structure of any phenomenon can be described in various ways, depending on which of its features are prioritized. The same is true for the phenomenon of uncertainty: Scholars from diverse disciplines have developed a variety of conceptual models and frameworks that prioritize different features. These various models and frameworks are neither "correct" nor "incorrect," but rather more or less useful; they are simply alternative ways of representing uncertainty in order to achieve some practical goal.

The practical goal of the current effort is to enable clinicians and patients to better manage and tolerate the variety of uncertainties they experience as they face medical problems. Toward this end, any description of the anatomy of uncertainty must account for the range of uncertainties that arise in medical care. It must also make pragmatic, actionable distinctions that can help clinicians and patients organize their approach to these uncertainties. With these objectives in mind, I now review existing conceptual frameworks that have been put forth to describe uncertainty in both medicine and science more broadly, and evaluate their strengths and weaknesses. I propose an

Uncertainty in Medicine. Paul K.J. Han, Oxford University Press. © Oxford University Press 2021.
DOI: 10.1093/oso/9780190270582.003.0003

alternative, integrative framework that describes medical uncertainty in terms of three organizing principles: source, issue, and locus. This three-dimensional conceptual framework lends a particular anatomical shape and form to the problem of medical uncertainty, which can help clinicians and patients evaluate and manage the variety of uncertainties that they experience in medicine.

CONCEPTUAL FRAMEWORKS OF MEDICAL UNCERTAINTY

The effort to develop a conceptual framework of medical uncertainty is by no means new. In her seminal ethnographic studies of uncertainty in medical training in the 1950s, sociologist Renée Fox developed a useful framework that identified three major types of uncertainty faced by physician-trainees in their efforts to achieve competence: (1) uncertainty arising from limitations in one's own (personal) medical knowledge; (2) uncertainty arising from limitations in the collective knowledge of the medical profession as a whole; and (3) a higher, metalevel uncertainty arising from the inability to distinguish between limitations in one's personal knowledge and those of the medical profession.[2] Fox's work was the first to identify and highlight the importance of this third, metalevel uncertainty and the inability to resolve it—that is, to diagnose the source of one's uncertainty—in the experience of physician-trainees.

Other researchers have since put forth frameworks that identify additional sources and types of uncertainty in medicine. Nursing scholar Merle Mishel developed a taxonomy of "uncertainty in illness" that identifies four distinct dimensions of uncertainty: (1) ambiguity, patients' self-evaluation of the state of illness as vague or unclear; (2) complexity, the multiplicity of varied cues patients perceive about treatment and the system of care; (3) deficient information, inadequate information concerning patients' diagnosis; and (4) unpredictability, absence of stability in the course of patients' illness and outcomes. Health communication scholar Austin Babrow has developed a more expansive taxonomy that includes five principal types and sources of uncertainty in healthcare: (1) complexity, arising from the multicausality, contingency, reciprocity, or unpredictability of a phenomenon; (2) qualities of information, its clarity, accuracy, completeness, volume, ambiguity, consistency, applicability, or trustworthiness; (3) probability, referring to one's belief in a specific probability or a range of probabilities; (4) structure of information, its order or integration; and (5) lay epistemology, people's own beliefs about a phenomenon. At a higher analytic level, Eric Beresford has identified three broad types of uncertainty in healthcare: technical, personal, and conceptual. Technical uncertainty results from "the paucity of adequate data to predict the effects of certain factors in the progress of a disease or the outcomes of certain interventions" (p. 7). Personal uncertainty is "rooted in the physician-patient relationship" (e.g., from the "lack of knowledge of the patient's values and concerns" or from clinicians' "sense of attachment" to patients). Conceptual uncertainty arises from the "problem of incommensurability and that of applying abstract criteria to concrete situations"; examples include the applicability of clinical practice guidelines to the case of an individual patient.

CONCEPTUAL FRAMEWORKS OF SCIENTIFIC UNCERTAINTY

Also relevant to the development of a framework of medical uncertainty are various conceptual frameworks of scientific uncertainty, developed by scholars in other disciplines. In engineering and risk analysis, for example, several frameworks have been developed to classify scientific uncertainties in statistical modeling. These frameworks make a useful conceptual distinction between "parameter uncertainty" (lack of knowledge about the values of a model's parameters) and "model uncertainty" (lack of knowledge needed to determine the correct scientific theory on which to base a model).[3,4] They also distinguish between "stochastic" and "epistemic" uncertainty.[5,6] Stochastic uncertainty pertains to the parameters of a risk model, originates from sampling or measurement error, and is mathematically expressible (e.g., using confidence intervals or probability density functions). Epistemic uncertainty, in contrast, reflects limitations in the current "state of knowledge" underlying models themselves, originates from competing theories or models, is difficult to quantify, and is manifest by subjective confusion or indecision.

One framework put forth by engineering and public policy scholar Granger Morgan has more specifically classified model-related uncertainty according to seven specific sources: (1) statistical variation arising from random measurement error; (2) subjective judgment due to systematic measurement error; (3) linguistic imprecision in the representation of quantities; (4) variability occurring naturally in a measured quantity over time or space; (5) inherent randomness and unpredictability arising from the indeterminacy (either real or apparent) of a phenomenon; (6) disagreement in interpretations of scientific evidence; and (7) approximation due to limitations in the capacity of a model to represent real-world systems. Biostatistician David Spiegelhalter has distinguished five objects and corresponding sources of uncertainty pertaining to risk modeling and analyses: (1) uncertainty regarding future events, arising from their essential unpredictability; (2) uncertainty about model parameters, arising from limitations in information; (3) uncertainty about model structures, arising from limitations in formalized knowledge; (4) uncertainties about known model inadequacies, arising from indeterminacy due to acknowledged limitations in understanding and modeling ability;

(5) uncertainties about unknown model adequacies, arising from ignorance or unknown limitations in knowledge.

Focusing more broadly on the scientific reasoning process, legal scholar Vern Walker has developed a taxonomy that distinguishes six main types of uncertainty: (1) conceptual, related to the definition and choice of descriptive concepts or variables; (2) measurement, involving the application of concepts or variables to specific, individual cases; (3) sampling, involving the generalization from specific, observed cases to unobserved cases; (4) modeling, involving the prediction of one predicate or variable as a mathematical function of other predicates or variables; (5) causal, involving the inference from certain mathematical functions between variables to conclusions about causal relationships; and (6) epistemic, involving the choice of interpretations for fundamental, logical concepts used throughout all levels.

Philosopher Silvio Funtowicz and colleagues have developed another broad conceptual taxonomy of uncertainty in science, known as "NUSAP" (numeral, unit, spread, assessment, and pedigree), aimed at informing policy initiatives to communicate and manage uncertainty. The foundation of this taxonomy is a definition of uncertainty as a situation of inadequate information of three main types: inexactness, unreliability, and ignorance.[7] The taxonomy classifies uncertainty along three primary dimensions: *location* (where the uncertainty manifests itself within a model of a natural phenomenon); *level* (where the uncertainty manifests itself along the spectrum between deterministic knowledge and total ignorance); and *nature* (whether the uncertainty is due to the imperfection of our knowledge or the inherent variability of the phenomenon being described).[8] The taxonomy further classifies each of these dimensions into more specific categories. The dimension of *location*, in turn, is further subdivided into context, model uncertainty, inputs, parameter uncertainty, and model outcome uncertainty. *Level* is subdivided into statistical (quantitatively described) uncertainty, "scenario" (qualitatively described) uncertainty, "recognised ignorance" (fundamental uncertainty about the mechanisms and functional relationships being studied), and "total ignorance." Finally, *nature* is subdivided into epistemic uncertainty (due to imperfect knowledge) and "variability uncertainty" (due to inherent variability). The last is often referred to as aleatory or ontological uncertainty, which arises from fundamental aspects of reality itself—specifically, indeterminacy or randomness in natural processes—as opposed to epistemic or epistemological uncertainty, which arises from limits in human knowledge of reality.

Perhaps the broadest, most comprehensive conceptual framework of scientific uncertainty is sociologist Michael Smithson's "taxonomy of ignorance," which catalogues a wide variety of types and sources of ignorance, or lack of knowledge. Smithson's taxonomy describes two major types and sources of ignorance: error (lack of knowledge due to distortion or incompleteness) and irrelevance (lack of knowledge due to deliberate or nondeliberate inattention). These two major forms of ignorance are further subdivided according to their sources. Error, for example, is subdivided into distortion and incompleteness, while irrelevance is subdivided into untopicality, taboo, and undecidability. Incompleteness of knowledge is further subdivided into uncertainty and absence of information. Smithson's taxonomy thus departs from our analysis in conceptualizing uncertainty as a specific subtype of ignorance consisting of incompleteness of knowledge and arising from more elemental sources: vagueness (presence of a range of possible values), probability (contingency on chance), or ambiguity (presence of multiple distinct possibilities). "Vagueness," in turn, arises from more fundamental sources, including "fuzziness" (lack of fine-graded distinctions or boundaries) and "nonspecificity" (imprecision of information), whereas "ambiguity" arises from information that is conflicting or subject to multiple interpretations.

INTEGRATING FRAMEWORKS

Existing frameworks of uncertainty in medicine and science demonstrate the rich and diverse ways in which uncertainty can be classified. These frameworks describe the anatomy of uncertainty by focusing on different features of the phenomenon. Some focus on the sources or causes of ignorance, others on its issues or objects—that is, the particular problem or aspect of reality about which one is ignorant. Still other frameworks focus on the particular parties or stakeholders who experience uncertainty (e.g., medical trainee vs. expert, medical science as a whole). The varying focus, breadth, and level of abstraction of these frameworks reflect the varying goals of their developers.

For the goal of helping clinicians and patients manage and tolerate uncertainty in medicine, existing conceptual frameworks provide a valuable foundation, but are also inadequate in several ways. Some are too narrow; they fail to capture the full range of causes or manifestations of medical uncertainty. Taxonomies of scientific uncertainty, for example, do not address the myriad practical and personal uncertainties clinicians and patients experience. Meanwhile, broad taxonomies such as Smithson's identify uncertainties (e.g., irrelevance and its subtypes of untopicality, taboo, and undecidability) that have limited relevance for routine clinical care. Still other taxonomies, such as Beresford's three-part classification (technical vs. personal vs. conceptual), are situated at a level of abstraction that is arguably too high to be practically useful.

Furthermore, existing uncertainty frameworks lack conceptual precision and coherence. Some pose distinctions that are not mutually exclusive. Examples include the distinction between ambiguity and deficient information in the healthcare-focused taxonomy of Mishel, between quality and structure of information in the taxonomy of Babrow, and between statistical, scenario, and recognized ignorance in the taxonomy of the NUSAP investigators. Other taxonomies combine conceptually distinct types of uncertainty within single categories while ignoring other important distinctions. For example, most taxonomies do not clearly distinguish between ignorance (lack of knowledge) as opposed to uncertainty (lack of awareness of one's ignorance) or between aleatory (or ontological) uncertainty arising from the nature of reality versus epistemic (or epistemological) uncertainty arising from information or human cognitive processes.

These problems raise the need for an integrative framework that is both broad enough to include the full range of important uncertainties that arise in medicine and narrow enough to focus on issues that are most relevant to clinicians and patients. The framework should ideally not only synthesize insights from other conceptual frameworks, but also facilitate practical actions that clinicians and patients can take to better manage and tolerate the uncertainties they face. In the remainder of this chapter, I attempt to develop an initial prototype of such a framework.

THE ANATOMY OF MEDICAL UNCERTAINTY: A THREE-DIMENSIONAL FRAMEWORK

This multidimensional, integrative framework prioritizes three features of medical uncertainty as organizing principles: its source (ultimate origin or cause), issue (substantive content or topical focus), and locus (the persons in whose minds uncertainty resides). The common-sense rationale for this approach is that all uncertainties in medicine come from somewhere, are about something, and are subjectively experienced by someone. These three features of uncertainty impart a logically coherent structure upon the phenomenon of uncertainty and a useful way of classifying the various uncertainties that arise in medicine, which can ultimately help clinicians and patients take a more organized approach to evaluating and managing them.

DIMENSION 1: SOURCES OF UNCERTAINTY

The first dimension, *source*, consists of the origins of uncertainty, which can be conceived at two interconnected levels: (1) a proximate, superficial, informational level consisting of the symbolic representations of ignorance (the stimuli that engender uncertainty when encountered by individuals); and (2) an ultimate, deeper, conceptual level consisting of the root causes of ignorance (the actual sources of the knowledge deficits that constitute the objects of uncertainty, but that normally remain latent and unacknowledged by individuals). Figure 3.1 depicts the sources of uncertainty at these two levels. At the superficial, informational level (upper part of the figure, in light

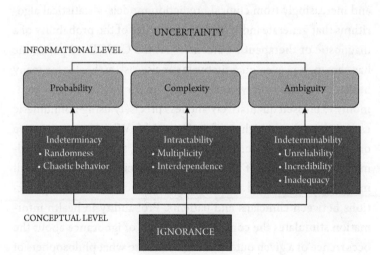

Figure 3.1 Sources of uncertainty.

gray) are three proximate sources of uncertainty: probability, complexity, and ambiguity.[9] At the deeper, conceptual level (lower part of the figure, in dark gray) are three corresponding ultimate root causes of ignorance: indeterminacy, intractability, and indeterminability.

Probability. Probability, otherwise known as *risk*, is a primary source of uncertainty in medicine and other important realms of life and a symbolic representation of uncertainty about the existence or occurrence of some unknown current or future event. The *Merriam-Webster Dictionary* defines probability as "the chance that a given event will occur" and "the ratio of the number of outcomes in an exhaustive set of equally likely outcomes that produce a given event to the total number of possible outcomes."[10] In medicine, probability is represented quantitatively through numeric estimates of various risks (e.g., the risk of having a positive SARS-CoV-2 [severe acute respiratory syndrome coronavirus 2] test result or of dying from COVID-19). Such evidence-based, "objective" probabilities are derived from empirical observations of the frequency of a given health outcome in a study population and increasingly from clinical prediction models—statistical algorithms that generate individualized estimates of the probability of a diagnostic or therapeutic outcome.[11] As the COVID-19 pandemic has shown, however, quantitatively precise risk estimates for many health outcomes simply do not exist, and probability is thus commonly expressed qualitatively and less precisely using nonnumeric estimates such as "high risk" or "low risk." Whether quantitative or qualitative, precise or imprecise, however, probability is the primary representation of uncertainty in medicine—the basis for all medical decisions and the common currency of clinical interactions between clinicians and patients. Probability in health information stimulates the conscious awareness of ignorance about the occurrence of a given outcome. It gives rise to what philosophers of statistics have termed *aleatory*, or *first-order* uncertainty—a specific subtype of uncertainty pertaining to the unpredictability of a given event.[12,13]

At a deeper, conceptual rather than informational level, probability manifests ignorance arising from the root cause of *indeterminacy*—the lack of a definitive or fixed outcome or result. This indeterminacy, in turn, arises from more fundamental sources. One source is the inherent *randomness* of natural processes, which makes future states fundamentally unknowable. The idea of randomness as an inherent property of natural processes has long been a controversial issue. It undermines modern science's foundational belief in determinism—the premise that natural processes are necessary consequences of prior events that operate through consistent, discoverable laws. This premise has been challenged, however, by scientific advances in fields ranging from quantum physics to evolutionary biology, which have posited inherent randomness in natural processes ranging from the movement of subatomic particles or waves to the production and transmission of genetic alterations in individuals and populations.[14–17] Inherent randomness in molecular processes may account for not only the evolutionary origin of the SARS-CoV-2 virus and its transmission from bats to humans, but also the host response of individuals to viral exposure and to therapeutic interventions for manifest COVID-19 disease.

Whether randomness truly exists or is merely apparent—reflecting human ignorance and the existence of unmeasured or "hidden variables," as Einstein claimed[18]—is a matter of continued debate. But natural processes need not be truly random to be indeterminate. Chaos theory has put forth the idea that natural processes can be deterministic, yet fundamentally indeterminate. They exhibit chaotic behavior due to several characteristic features: nonlinear dynamics (multiplicative or irregular patterns of response), feedback (the direct and indirect influence of a phenomenon's effects on its causes), and extreme sensitivity to initial conditions (the potential for very small errors in mathematical modeling efforts to produce exponentially large errors in predictions).[19-23] These are defining features of "complex adaptive systems"—collections of individual phenomena that interact in multiple ways.[24] Chaotic behavior makes it impossible to precisely predict the course of the COVID-19 pandemic at the population level or the outcomes of COVID-19 illness at the individual level. As systems scientists Reuben McDaniel and Dean Driebe argued, chaotic behavior is part of the natural order of the universe, and cannot be avoided, eliminated, or controlled.[20,25] In other words, indeterminacy is ultimately ontological in nature—rooted in the basic structures of reality—and fundamentally irreducible (Figure 3.1).

Ambiguity. The second major source of uncertainty, ambiguity, was first described in 1921 by economist Frank Knight[26] and formalized in 1961 in seminal work by decision theorist Daniel Ellsberg.[27] Ellsberg used the term *ambiguity* to signify a particular feature of risk information: "a quality depending on the amount, type, reliability, and 'unanimity,' of information, and giving rise to one's degree of 'confidence' in an estimate of relative likelihood" (p. 644). Ambiguity is high "when there are questions of reliability and relevance of information, and particularly where there is conflicting opinion and evidence," and Ellsberg showed that it has important effects on human judgment and decision-making. Specifically, when people are confronted by ambiguity they form pessimistic appraisals of risks and avoid decision-making—a response that has come to be known as *ambiguity aversion.*[27,28] Ellsberg thus deduced that "there are uncertainties that are not risks"—that people base risky decisions on not only the probability of a given choice outcome, but also the "nature of one's information" about this probability (p. 643).

In medicine, ambiguity is often expressed quantitatively through risk ranges or confidence intervals around probabilities (e.g., 71%–98% estimated sensitivity of SARS-CoV-2 testing or a 0.2%–1%

population-wide COVID-19 mortality rate). As the COVID-19 pandemic has demonstrated, however, precise probability estimates for various health outcomes are typically lacking, and risks are truly unknown; ambiguity is thus more often expressed qualitatively using hedging language (e.g., "approximately," "roughly," "our best guess"). Ambiguity in health information stimulates conscious awareness of ignorance about the quality of evidence regarding the occurrence of a given outcome. It thus gives rise to what philosophers of statistics have termed *epistemic,* or *second-order* uncertainty—that is, uncertainty about probability.[28]

At the deeper, conceptual rather than informational level, ambiguity manifests ignorance arising from the root cause of *indeterminability*—the inability to establish a definitive or fixed outcome, result, or answer. As a source of ignorance, indeterminability is squarely epistemological (rooted in human knowledge of reality) as opposed to ontological (rooted in the basic structures of reality) (Figure 3.1). It arises from more fundamental sources that Ellsberg identified: *unreliability, incredibility,* and *inadequacy.* *Unreliability* refers to shortcomings in the consistency and robustness of medical knowledge, which originates from limitations in empirical evidence and the methods used to analyze it.[29] In the COVID-19 pandemic, manifestations of unreliability include varying estimates of the accuracy of different SARS-CoV-2 diagnostic tests. *Incredibility* refers to shortcomings in the trustworthiness or believability of medical knowledge, which originates from various factors, including interpretive biases that lead to conflicting interpretations.[30] Manifestations include contradictory guidance on mask use put forth by various government officials and health experts. *Inadequacy* refers to shortcomings in the amount of medical knowledge itself, which results from missing data or unmeasured variables. Manifestations of inadequacy include the lack of existing information on the effectiveness of SARS-CoV-2 vaccines and COVID-19 treatments that are currently being developed and evaluated in clinical trials.

In theory, the unreliability, incredibility, and inadequacy of medical knowledge can be mitigated through the acquisition of more or better evidence; indeterminability is thus a reducible cause of ignorance. This is the premise of the entire enterprise of medical research and evidence-based medicine. It is also the aspirational goal of the application of "big data" and predictive analytic technologies, including machine learning and artificial intelligence, to health are problems. An important exception, however, is indeterminability regarding the true probability of any single event—such as whether any individual patient exposed to the SARS-CoV-2 virus will become infected, have a positive diagnostic test result, develop symptomatic disease, respond to treatment, or subsequently die from COVID-19. From a practical standpoint, single-event probabilities are indeterminable due to methodological problems that prevent all causal variables that determine an event's occurrence from being accounted for.

From a more fundamental, theoretical standpoint, however, single-event probabilities are indeterminable due to logical problems inherent to the notion of probability itself. In medicine and all other realms of our lives, probabilities are derived from—and expressed in terms of—the retrospectively observed frequencies of events repeated in either time (over the long run) or space (across a given population of individuals). The problem, however, is that these objective probabilities are inapplicable to single events experienced by individuals.[31,32] It makes sense to say that an individual who tosses a coin repeatedly will obtain a heads 50% of the time, or that a population of seriously ill COVID-19 patients treated with dexamethasone have a 28-day mortality rate of 29%. However, these numbers have no literal, logically coherent meaning for any single coin toss or individual life: the coin will land on either heads or tails, the person will either live or die. As philosopher Ian Hacking observed, "It does not make sense to speak of the 'frequency' of a single event."[31] Statistician Bruno de Finetti thus famously declared that, "Probability does not exist,"[33] meaning that at the individual, single-event level, probabilities are not objective facts but subjective beliefs with no single "true" value.[31,32] In other words, even the most precise, evidence-based probabilities in medicine—and all endeavors of human life—are fundamentally ambiguous (unknown): when applied to single events experienced by individuals, their true magnitude is indeterminable.

Complexity. The third major source of uncertainty, complexity, refers to features of information that make it difficult to understand. Complexity is an emergent property of medical information; unlike probability and ambiguity, it is not intentionally represented and actively conveyed, but emergent and passively perceived. Complexity arises when informational elements increase in number, variety, or interconnectedness. The prognosis of COVID-19, for example, is known to depend on multiple factors (e.g., sociodemographic characteristics such as age and race, comorbidities such as diabetes mellitus and pulmonary disease), and the significant unexplained variability in the survival of individual patients suggests the influence of many more unmeasured variables that interact in myriad ways. Informational complexity stimulates the conscious awareness of ignorance about whether a given problem can be adequately understood, and thereby gives rise to epistemic uncertainty.

At the deeper, conceptual rather than informational level, complexity manifests ignorance arising from the root cause of *intractability*—the resistance of a problem to human comprehension and control. Intractability, in turn, arises from two more fundamental sources (Figure 3.1). The first is *multiplicity* in the components, attributes, or implications of a given problem; examples include the existence of numerous disease risk factors, diagnostic possibilities, therapeutic alternatives, or health outcomes. The second key source of intractability is *interdependence* between the components of a problem; examples include the existence of moderating or mediating relationships between causal variables (e.g., gene-by-environment interactions) or conditional relationships between different outcomes.[19,20] Importantly, multiplicity and interdependence are both objective and subjective in nature; they depend on both the actual and perceived number and connectedness of elements comprising a given problem. Multiplicity and interdependence, for example, are undisputed, objective properties of the spread of the COVID-19 pandemic. Yet the extent to which these properties are subjectively perceived—and to which the spread of COVID-19 is consequently deemed an intractable problem and object of ignorance—can vary among individuals depending on their own capacity for handling complexity. Laypersons, physicians, and statistical modelers will have different views on these issues.

Among the primary sources of ignorance, intractability is thus situated in between indeterminacy and indeterminability; its essential features overlap conceptually with both (Figure 3.1). Like indeterminacy, intractability is ontological (rooted in the basic structures of reality) and thus irreducible; like indeterminability, however, it is epistemological (rooted in human knowledge) and thus reducible. Advances in computer technologies have enabled many previously intractable problems to be solved, and recent advances, including artificial intelligence and quantum computing, are making many more problems tractable. By extending the capacity of the human mind to deal with multiplicity and interdependence, these technologies are reducing the complexity of many problems.

Overlapping concepts. The two-level framework of sources of uncertainty makes logical distinctions between different sources of both uncertainty (probability, ambiguity, and complexity) and ignorance (indeterminacy, indeterminability, and intractability). However, the conceptual boundaries between these sources are not definite or fixed. Granger Morgan, for example, has aptly questioned the distinction between probability and ambiguity, arguing that it rests on a mistaken belief that a single "true" probability exists in the first place.[34] Without this belief, the distinction between probability and ambiguity collapses: ambiguity (i.e., informational unreliability, incredibility, or inadequacy) becomes an inseparable part of all probabilities, and epistemic (second-order) uncertainty reduces to aleatory (first-order) uncertainty. Probability estimates themselves simply become symbolic representations of uncertainty arising from any and all of these sources. In a similar vein, one can also question the conceptual distinctions between indeterminacy, indeterminability, and intractability. From a logical standpoint, a phenomenon that is either indeterminable or intractable, for example, must also be indeterminate.

Yet conceptual overlap between the various sources of uncertainty and ignorance represented in the current model does not undermine the value of distinguishing between them. Although the distinction between probability and ambiguity may have questionable normative validity, it has unquestionable descriptive validity; it accurately reflects how people think and act in response to uncertainty. The well-documented phenomenon of ambiguity aversion has established that ambiguity has independent, additive effects on judgments and decisions, over and above probability. In other words, ambiguity exists and matters to people, irrespective of whether it should.[35]

Furthermore, although some sources of uncertainty and ignorance may not be mutually exclusive, distinguishing between them can help clinicians and patients account for all potentially important and addressable sources in a given situation. For example, complexity (intractability) is arguably an important source of uncertainty in most medical situations—even when the primary source is probability (indeterminacy) or ambiguity (indeterminability). Complexity is an even more important source of uncertainty for persons with low health literacy or numeracy. Regardless of what actions are taken to address the primary sources of uncertainty in these situations, therefore, an appropriate additional response is to enact efforts to reduce complexity (e.g., simplifying, breaking down, and organizing information in a way that clarifies its gist meaning).[36,37] From a practical standpoint, the conceptual overlap between different sources of uncertainty thus matters little; distinguishing between these sources still serves the useful purpose of allowing clinicians and patients to be aware of their unique contribution to the uncertainty at hand and to enact appropriate measures to address them.

DIMENSION 2: ISSUES OF UNCERTAINTY

The three primary *sources* of uncertainty (probability, complexity, ambiguity) are the superficial, informational manifestations of ignorance arising from deeper conceptual causes (indeterminacy, intractability, indeterminability). But these sources of uncertainty are themselves manifest through a variety of substantive *issues*—that is, specific, concrete problems, outcomes, situations, or alternatives that represent the objects of one's ignorance. These issues constitute the second dimension of uncertainty and fall into three main categories: scientific, practical, and personal (Figure 3.2).[9] Broadly speaking, scientific uncertainty is disease centered, whereas practical and personal uncertainties are system and patient centered.

Scientific. Scientific uncertainty in medicine focuses on four main issues of medical problems: diagnosis, prognosis, cause, and treatment. *Diagnosis*—the specific identity of the problem at hand—is the primary issue that prompts many patients to seek medical care in the first place. Answering the question "What is wrong?" is the first order of business for both patients and clinicians. For the young mother seeking evaluation for new-onset

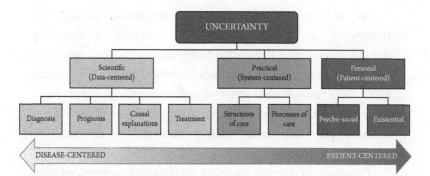

Figure 3.2 Issues of uncertainty in healthcare.

cough, fatigue, and fever, the main issue is to determine the diagnosis for her symptoms, and her initial medical evaluation focuses on resolving this issue. *Prognosis* is another critical issue. "What will happen to me?" is the next question that arises whether or not a firm diagnosis is made. For the young mother with newly diagnosed COVID-19, the main issue is to determine her expected response to treatment and her risk of death or other adverse clinical outcomes. Her subsequent clinical evaluation is directed toward resolving this issue using radiographic studies, measures of blood oxygen and other biomarkers, and clinical prediction models. *Cause* is another critical issue of uncertainty. "Why is this problem happening?" is a key question that affects how people respond to medical problems. For the members of the general public who are being asked to adhere to social distancing and mask use, the main issue is to understand what causes the SARS-CoV-2 virus to spread and why these risk-reducing measures work. *Treatment* is the final important issue for both patients and clinicians. "What should be done to cure or manage this medical problem?" is the question to which all others lead. For the young mother with COVID-19, the main issue is to determine what she needs to do to get through her illness and to move ahead with her life.

All of these issues—diagnostic, prognostic, causal, and therapeutic—are disease centered and "scientific" in that they depend on empirical knowledge and evidence collected systematically using the theories and methods of medical science. Uncertainty about these various issues arises when this knowledge and evidence are insufficient and when ignorance arising from any of the sources described previously (indeterminacy, intractability, indeterminability) cannot be reduced.

Practical. Yet scientific issues are not the only important, substantive objects of uncertainty in medicine. Practical issues—pertaining to the structures and processes of healthcare—are equally important and encompass the various procedures and actions that patients and clinicians must undertake to receive and provide medical care. For our young patient with COVID-19, these issues include the competence and trustworthiness of her healthcare providers and the healthcare system as a whole and her ability to pay for her care. Other important practical issues include how to get to a healthcare facility, make an appointment to see a healthcare provider and receive needed services (e.g., diagnostic testing for SARS-CoV-2 virus infection, treatment for COVID-19, follow-up care), pay for care, and deal with health insurance issues. The tremendous growth in recent years of patient navigation programs for cancer and other diseases attests to the importance of practical uncertainties. For clinicians, practical issues of uncertainty include patients' ability to understand their illnesses and to adhere to medical recommendations. During the COVID-19 pandemic, other important practical uncertainties for clinicians have included the adequacy of existing procedures and protocols for preventing the spread of infection in healthcare facilities and the availability of personal protective equipment.

These and other issues pertaining to the structures and processes of care are "practical" in the sense that they are system-centered, focused on healthcare delivery processes, and resolvable through trial and error. In recent years, however, practical uncertainties have become scientific as healthcare safety and quality have become an increasing focus of both system improvement initiatives and medical research.

Personal. A final important category of issues that represent important objects of uncertainty in medicine is personal—that is, pertaining to psychosocial, economic, and existential concerns of both patients and clinicians. For our young mother with COVID-19, personal issues of uncertainty extend well beyond scientific concerns about her diagnosis, prognosis, and treatment or practical concerns about what she needs to do to obtain the medical care she needs. This patient's issues of uncertainty encompass equally important concerns about how her illness will affect her ability to care for her children, to work and make an income, and to spend time with loved ones, including her 80-year-old father, who has advanced Alzheimer dementia and lives in a nursing home. Her personal uncertainties also encompass the greatest mysteries of all: the meaning of life and death, being and nonbeing, and the purpose of her own existence.

Personal issues are important objects of uncertainty for clinicians as well as patients and also encompass moral and existential concerns. For the 45-year-old critical care physician working in New York City at the height of the COVID-19 pandemic, personal issues of uncertainty include whether to commit intensive care unit beds, ventilators, and other scarce medical resources to patients like the previously healthy young mother with severe COVID-19 pneumonia, as opposed to others like her elderly father with dementia and chronic obstructive pulmonary disease. But the physician's moral uncertainties are even more personal. Every day she goes to work she risks becoming infected, while every night she returns home she risks spreading infection to her family. Every day the physician on the clinical front line must therefore make additional value judgments and morally distressing personal choices: between promoting the well-being of her patients or protecting the well-being of her family, between isolating herself away from home or exposing her loved ones to the possibility of infection, between continuing her work or not. These difficult choices, along with the randomness and sheer magnitude of suffering and death she encounters on a daily basis, challenge the physician's sense of meaning and purpose in life. They become issues of existential uncertainty that deal with the most profound "metaquestions"—as Renée Fox aptly labeled them—about the reasons for pain, suffering, and death, and the meaning and finitude of life.[38]

All of these issues are personal—as opposed to scientific or practical—in the sense that they are patient or clinician centered, focused on fundamental human values and questions of meaning, and not resolvable through either trial and error or the acquisition of additional scientific evidence. The COVID-19 crisis has demonstrated, furthermore, how uncertainties about such personal issues can cause just as much human suffering—for both patients and clinicians—as uncertainties about any of the strictly scientific issues that arise in medicine. They generate moral distress, existential anxiety, and burnout among patients and clinicians alike, although they have historically been unaddressed in medicine. In recent years, however, various trends in healthcare—including a growing emphasis on patient-centered care as well as provider well-being—have focused attention on these personal issues of uncertainty and stimulated greater efforts to address them.

DIMENSION 3: LOCUS OF UNCERTAINTY

The third and final dimension of uncertainty consists of its *locus*—that is, the person or persons in whose minds uncertainty—as the conscious metacognitive awareness of ignorance—resides. As the

COVID-19 crisis has shown, medical uncertainty can reside in the minds of any number of people: patients, clinicians, researchers, administrators, policymakers, government officials, the general public. The precise locus of uncertainty depends on several factors: prior knowledge, experience, and exposure to information; concerns that make different uncertainties more or less salient to different persons; and interpersonal interactions that transmit knowledge and produce a shared consciousness of ignorance.

This dynamic is illustrated in Figure 3.3, which depicts the locus of uncertainty between just two parties, a clinician and a patient. In some situations, both parties reside in a state of "mutual ignorance"— that is, lacking not only knowledge about a given medical problem, but also awareness of their lack of knowledge (lower right-hand box). In situations of "unilateral uncertainty," in contrast, one party resides in a state of ignorance, the other in a state of uncertainty— that is, consciously aware of his or her ignorance (lower left-hand and upper right-hand boxes). This asymmetric, unshared uncertainty is manifested clinically when either the clinician is aware of scientific ignorance about a particular scientific issue (e.g., the effectiveness of monoclonal antibody therapy for early COVID-19 disease) and the

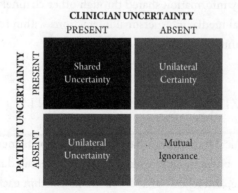

Figure 3.3 Locus of uncertainty: clinician and patient.

patient is not, or else the patient is aware of ignorance about a particular personal issue (e.g., her family's ability to cope with her illness, both psychologically and financially) and the physician is not.

In other situations, clinicians and patients reside in a state of shared uncertainty—equally aware (uncertain) of what they do not know about important issues of mutual concern (upper left-hand box). Such symmetric, shared uncertainty is the ultimate goal of shared decision-making (SDM), an idealized process of care that promotes patient autonomy by facilitating the bidirectional transfer of information between clinicians and patients. As discussed in Chapter 2, this process involves the exchange of explanatory models and the co-construction of a body of knowledge and a shared consciousness of what is known. But it also involves the co-construction of a body of ignorance and a shared consciousness of what is not known; SDM ultimately promotes shared uncertainty among patients and clinicians. The collective impact of SDM on medical uncertainty, however, is so far minimal given that SDM is not yet the norm in medical practice, and patient-clinician interactions are a limited source of medical information for most laypersons. As the COVID-19 pandemic has illustrated, much of the medical uncertainty experienced by patients and members of the general public is generated by information shared through other channels (e.g., mass media, social media, interpersonal interactions within social groups and communities).

VISUALIZING MEDICAL UNCERTAINTY

The anatomical framework I have presented depicts medical uncertainty as a phenomenon with three fundamental dimensions—source, issue, and locus—that are immanent within each other. For any given uncertainty about any of the substantive issues (scientific, practical, or personal) that comprise the second dimension of the framework, the underlying cause may be any of the proximate, informational sources (probability, ambiguity, complexity) or ultimate, conceptual sources (indeterminacy, indeterminability, intractability) that comprise the first dimension. Any or all of these sources may generate uncertainty about not only the diagnosis, prognosis, cause, and treatment of a given medical condition (scientific uncertainty), but also the procedures required to access healthcare or the expected quality of one's care (practical uncertainty) and the effects of one's medical condition or treatment on one's personal relationships, goals, and sense of purpose and meaning in life (personal uncertainty). The young mother with COVID-19, for example, may experience uncertainty about numerous issues: her chances of recovery and survival with and without various treatments; the availability of effective treatments; the competence of her physician and clinical care team; the impact of her illness on her ability to both care for her children and maintain her family's financial well-being. In theory, probabilities exist for all of these outcomes; however, these probabilities are unknown (i.e., ambiguous) in varying degrees, and the uncertainty they generate is further compounded by varying degrees of complexity. Furthermore, these and other uncertainties are unevenly distributed in the mind of the patient and of her physician; while some are shared by both parties, others reside exclusively in the mind of one party or another.

This three-dimensional framework is not the only way of visualizing medical uncertainty, and does not capture every potentially important aspect of the phenomenon. It simply imposes an artificial, theoretical structure on reality; its categories and constructs—like those of other frameworks—have no definite ontological grounding. However, the framework does capture important features of medical uncertainty and provides a practically useful navigational tool that can help clinicians and patients to evaluate and manage it in a more systematic, intentional manner. It gives a concrete form and shape to the problem, which can allow clinicians and patients to "see" what they are doing—to account for the variety of uncertainties that arise in different situations and to ensure that they are addressed. Toward this end, the potential utility of the framework is threefold, corresponding to each of the major dimensions of uncertainty.

First, by focusing attention on the source of uncertainty, the framework can help clinicians and patients clarify the prognosis— that is, the relative reducibility or irreducibility—of different uncertainties and the appropriate goals and strategies for managing them. For example, some uncertainties arising from complexity are theoretically reducible (e.g., information about the potential harms and side effects of medications), as are some uncertainties arising from ambiguity (e.g., low-quality observational evidence that emerged early in the COVID-19 pandemic and suggested that cigarette smoking had a protective effect). In cases such as these, the appropriate goal is to reduce uncertainty by improving the comprehensibility and coherence of information and correcting misconceptions. Strategies include not only simplifying and organizing information, as previously discussed, but also clarifying the quality of available empirical evidence.[36] In contrast, uncertainties arising from other sources are fundamentally irreducible and thus entail different goals and management strategies. These include uncertainties arising from both probability and ambiguity—whether pertaining to the onset of disease, the benefits and harms of medical treatment, or the practical or personal consequences of illness and its treatment. In these circumstances the proper goal is not to reduce but to increase and palliate uncertainty—that is, to help ameliorate its negative psychological effects. By clarifying the prognosis of uncertainty, the conceptual framework thus enables clinicians and patients to take a targeted, rather than a one-size-fits-all, approach to managing uncertainty and to have more realistic expectations about the outcomes of this effort.

Second, by focusing attention on the issue of uncertainty, the framework can promote greater attention to existing knowledge gaps and help clinicians and patients prioritize which gaps are most important to address. Informed decision-making and SDM require clinicians and patients to reach a mutual understanding of scientific uncertainties regarding the benefits and harms of medical interventions, as well as personal uncertainties regarding the values and preferences of patients. Yet the finite nature of human cognitive resources and the infinite demands of everyday life make it impossible to attend to every issue of potential uncertainty in medicine. Clinicians and patients need some way of prioritizing the issues of uncertainty that need to be addressed in any given situation, and a conceptual framework that classifies these issues can support this task.

Third, by focusing attention on the locus of uncertainty, the framework can promote greater attention to the uncertainties that matter most to patients as well as clinicians. A conceptual framework that identifies not only what uncertainties exist but also who is experiencing them can sensitize clinicians and patients to inequities in their relative awareness of ignorance and encourage them to engage with one another to reduce these inequities. A conceptual framework that helps clarify the locus of uncertainty can also heighten clinicians' and patients' awareness of interpersonal discrepancies in their relative tolerance of uncertainty—that is, their propensity toward positive versus negative psychological responses to the conscious awareness of ignorance.[39,40] It can help both parties understand how differences in their personal uncertainty tolerance may be influencing their medical judgments and decisions, experiences with care, and the quality of the clinician-patient relationship. It can help clinicians and patients to account for these differences and to prevent them from creating misunderstanding or conflict.

In all of these ways, a three-dimensional conceptual framework can facilitate a more intentional, targeted, and rational approach to evaluating and managing medical uncertainty. By providing a way of visualizing, ordering, and objectifying an otherwise invisible, disordered, subjective reality, it helps us to attain a higher vantage point—to "metaphorically climb a tree," as philosopher John Dewey put it[1]—from which we can exert greater control over our uncertainty and our various psychological responses to it. Before we can accomplish this goal, however, we need to develop a better understanding of these responses, and I now turn to this task.

Chapter 4

The Natural History of Uncertainty

The natural man dislikes the dis-ease which accompanies the doubtful and is ready to take almost any means to end it.

—John Dewey[1]

The evaluation and management of medical uncertainty, like any other medical problem, requires a thorough understanding of not only its nature, etiology, and anatomy but also its natural history— that is, how the problem evolves and what specific responses it elicits. A substantial body of empirical research has generated key insights on these responses; however, the challenge is that these insights have originated mostly outside of medicine and have not been integrated into a single coherent account. My goal in this chapter is to address this challenge by reviewing key insights on people's psychological responses to uncertainty and to integrate these insights with personal observations of clinicians' and patients' responses—derived from my own experience as a researcher, physician, and human being—to develop a provisional conceptual framework of the natural history of medical uncertainty. This framework categorizes responses to medical uncertainty into two main types: (1) *primary*, consisting of clinicians' and patients' initial cognitive, emotional, and behavioral responses to uncertainty; and (2) *secondary*, consisting of various compensatory strategies that clinicians and patients employ to regulate their primary responses to uncertainty (Figure 4.1).

Uncertainty in Medicine. Paul K.J. Han, Oxford University Press. © Oxford University Press 2021.
DOI: 10.1093/oso/9780190270582.003.0004

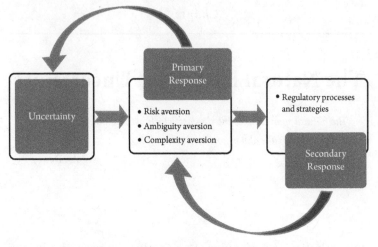

Figure 4.1 Natural history of medical uncertainty.

PRIMARY RESPONSES TO UNCERTAINTY: RISK, AMBIGUITY, AND COMPLEXITY AVERSION

A vast body of empirical research in various social science disciplines, ranging from anthropology to psychology to sociology, has consistently shown that uncertainty provokes a wide variety of primarily aversive psychological responses. Although uncertainty is a higher-level, metacognitive form of knowledge—a knowledge of our own ignorance—that serves adaptive functions, human beings generally dislike being in this state and will "take almost any means to end it," as Dewey observed.[1] Past research on people's cognitive, emotional, and behavioral responses to different types of uncertainty has identified three distinct, prototypical syndromes that share several important features: risk aversion, ambiguity aversion, and complexity aversion.

Risk aversion. The most well-documented syndrome, risk aversion, focuses specifically on psychological responses to uncertainty arising proximately from probability in information and ultimately from the indeterminacy of a given outcome (Chapter 3). The focus of a large body of research in behavioral economics and decision psychology, risk aversion is formally defined as the reluctance or hesitancy of decision-makers to choose risky prospects even when they involve greater expected gain.[2-5] Risk aversion is manifest by decision-makers' tendency to discount the value of uncertain versus certain gains and even to pay a premium to avoid such uncertainty. Such behavior represents a departure from rationality as defined by subjective expected utility theory, which holds that people should prefer choice options that maximize expected utility (defined as the product of the probability and the personal utility of a given outcome).

Risk aversion has been empirically demonstrated in numerous studies examining various problems and decisions, although its observed consistency and strength have been lower in real life than in laboratory settings and decisions not involving monetary gambles.[3,6] Risk aversion also depends on various attributes of the risky situation. One important attribute, described by psychologists Daniel Kahneman and Amos Tversky in their seminal Prospect Theory, is whether a given risky outcome represents a relative loss or gain compared to one's reference point.[7] People have been shown to be less risk averse (more risk taking) in the domain of losses than in the domain of gains; they judge the value of a risky choice option more favorably and are more apt to take a chance to avoid the prospect of loss.

Risk aversion, furthermore, has not only behavioral but also cognitive and emotional manifestations. Cognitive manifestations consist of subjective perceptions of vulnerability.[8] Psychologist Paul Slovic, in his "psychometric paradigm" of risk perception, has shown how these perceptions are determined by particular features of the threats at hand, including their known versus unknown nature and the sense of "dread" they evoke.[9] Emotional manifestations of risk aversion consist of negative affective states such as worry.[10] Clinical psychologists have conceptualized worry as a direct consequence of perceptions of risk and indeterminacy; Thomas Borkevic and colleagues have defined worry as a negative affective response produced by issues whose outcome is uncertain but contains the possibility of negative outcomes.[11] In a similar vein, Melissa Robichaud, Naomi Koerner, and Michel Dugas have characterized worry as an emotional sequela of "thinking about every possible outcome ahead of time."[12]

Ambiguity aversion. Another important syndrome of responses to uncertainty, ambiguity aversion, was originally described by Daniel Ellsberg in work previously discussed (Chapter 3). This syndrome consists of psychological responses to uncertainty arising proximately from ambiguity (lack of reliability, credibility, or adequacy) in information and ultimately from the indeterminability of a given outcome.[13] Ambiguity aversion has been a major focus of research in behavioral economics and decision psychology and has been defined as the tendency to avoid or defer decision-making when probabilities are ambiguous.[13-17] Like risk aversion, ambiguity aversion represents a departure from rational decision-making as defined by subjective expected utility theory. Ambiguity aversion manifests the dependency of decisions on not only the probability and personal utility of choice options but also a third factor: the quality of the information at hand—specifically, its perceived reliability, credibility, or adequacy.

Ambiguity aversion has been demonstrated in numerous studies to be a robust effect, persisting even when the odds strongly favor ambiguous options in choice scenarios.[13,16] Like risk aversion, however, the observed strength and consistency of ambiguity aversion have been lower in real-life settings than in games of chance in laboratory settings.[18-21] Ambiguity aversion depends on various situational characteristics, including whether losses or gains are at stake; people appear to be ambiguity seeking rather than ambiguity averse when confronted with the prospect of loss.[16,18,22] Other situational characteristics, such as the degree of existing ambiguity and the manner in which it is communicated, also appear to be influential.[16,23,24]

Like risk aversion, ambiguity aversion has not only behavioral but also cognitive and emotional manifestations. Ambiguity has been shown to promote not only deferral or avoidance of decision-making but also "alarmist" perceptions of vulnerability and pessimistic appraisals of risks and benefits,[25-27] as well as fear, worry, and anxiety.[23,28] Fear itself may represent a specific response to uncertainty arising from ambiguity as opposed to other sources of uncertainty. Clinical psychologist and researcher Nick Carleton has classified different types of fear within a hierarchical structure and argued that the most fundamental type is "fear of the unknown": a fundamental, primordial emotion consisting of "an individual's propensity to experience fear caused by the perceived *absence of information* at any level of consciousness or point of processing"[29] (italics mine). Carleton has further argued that "fear of the unknown may be a, or possibly the, fundamental fear" underlying numerous other higher-order fears, including fear of pain and even death. From this perspective, it is uncertainty arising specifically from the indeterminability of future events that is the root cause of fear as an fundamental emotional response.

Complexity aversion. The final important syndrome of psychological responses to uncertainty is known as complexity aversion. This set of responses focuses specifically on uncertainty arising proximately from complexity in information (features that make it difficult to understand) and ultimately from the intractability of a phenomenon and has been described in terms of both "complexity aversion" and "choice overload." Complexity aversion refers to a dislike of complexity and an avoidance of decision-making when the number or "compoundness" of choice options increases.[15,30] Choice overload refers to the tendency to stick to the default option in choice problems that contain multiple alternatives[31-33] and has been alternatively described as the overchoice effect, the tyranny of choice, and the too-much-choice effect.[33] Behavioral outcomes associated with choice overload include a decrease in both the motivation to choose and the strength of one's preferences and satisfaction with decision-making and an increase in negative emotions, including disappointment and regret.[34-37]

Complexity aversion has been demonstrated in controlled laboratory experiments as well as studies in naturalistic settings involving various problems. In one study in the medical domain, for example, the complexity introduced by adding choice options in a hypothetical medication-prescribing scenario led physicians to avoid decision-making altogether.[38] Past research has suggested, however, that the extent of complexity aversion varies and is likely moderated by numerous factors. These include the nature of the choice and trade-offs involved, the number of choice options and attributes, prior preferences, and environmental factors, including time pressure and decision support resources.[33] Cognitive and emotional manifestations of complexity aversion have been less well described, although existing evidence suggests that complexity may have negative effects not only on decision-making but also perceptions of decision satisfaction and the difficulty of decision-making.[33] More research is needed to understand the emotional effects of uncertainty arising from complexity and intractability.

SECONDARY RESPONSES TO UNCERTAINTY: REGULATORY PROCESSES AND STRATEGIES

The syndromes of probability, ambiguity, and complexity aversion demonstrate that irrespective of its specific sources, uncertainty provokes predominantly negative psychological responses. Cognitively, it engenders perceptions of vulnerability and pessimistic appraisals of risks and benefits. Emotionally it elicits feelings of fear, worry, and anxiety. Behaviorally, it promotes decision avoidance or defer-ral. The true extent and magnitude of these effects in medicine—and the relative strength of risk, ambiguity, and complexity aversion—is not known given that relatively few studies have investigated these phenomena in the medical domain. There is no reason to believe that these phenomena would not have equal or even greater effects in real, high-stakes medical situations; however, our knowledge of exactly how clinicians and patients respond to different uncertainties in medicine is currently incomplete.

This is all the more the case given the types of psychological responses that have been the focus of past research on uncertainty. Reflecting its overarching applied aim to improve decision-making, this research has focused primarily on understanding negative, inhib-itory effects of uncertainty on this outcome in particular. Much less attention, correspondingly, has been devoted to understanding its positive effects and on outcomes other than decision-making. Even less attention has been devoted to understanding people's secondary responses to uncertainty—that is, the compensatory strategies they use to cope with their negative primary responses.

I now attempt to bridge these knowledge gaps by drawing on various sources of evidence, including my own empirical research and clinical experiences, to develop a provisional conceptual frame-work that captures the breadth of clinicians' and patients' secondary responses to uncertainty. The framework organizes these responses according to their focus and goals.

THE CONCEPT OF REGULATION

A key organizing concept for this framework is the idea of "regula-tion." The term *regulate* originates from the Latin verb *regula*, mean-ing to "rule," and dictionaries offer other definitions (e.g., to "control or maintain the rate or speed of," to "govern or direct according to rule," to "bring order, method, or uniformity to," and to "fix or adjust the time, amount, degree, or rate of").[39] In these definitions, regulation signifies a dynamic process aimed at exerting control over some problem, and provides a useful concept for thinking about the fundamental psychological processes involved in people's secondary responses to uncertainty. Theories of "self-regulation," for example, explain how individuals exert control over themselves and their environment by altering their own responses or inner states.[40] Social psychologist Roy Baumeister and colleagues have defined self-regulation as a high-level executive function with several attributes, including reflexive awareness and transcendence—"the human capacity to process and respond to things or events that lie beyond the immediate stimulus environment"—as well as commitment to standards, monitoring of the self and its behaviors, and the capacity to adapt and make changes.[41] Self-regulation is thus the ultimate metacognitive activity: a process in which an "observing ego" monitors and reacts to its own states.[42] Self-regulation can be unconscious and automatic as well as conscious and deliberate and is thought to operate like a strength or energy that can become depleted when used or increased with regular exercise.[40] Self-regulation has been a key concept for understanding how people respond to various psychological states and demands, including emotions[42-44] as well as illness and other threats to health.[45,46]

The concept of self-regulation as a metacognitive activity provides a useful way of thinking about people's secondary responses to uncertainty. Uncertainty itself is a metacognitive state—a higher-level knowledge of one's ignorance—that serves various adaptive, regulatory functions that include inhibiting overconfidence and promoting caution, restraint, and prudence in decision-making. The paradox of the human condition, however, is that this same metacognitive state can be psychologically aversive and maladaptive. It can also promote underconfidence and inhibit decisive action in situations that call for it. For these reasons, both uncertainty and our various psychological responses to it ultimately require self-regulation at an even higher metacognitive level.

I now present a provisional conceptual taxonomy that describes some of the main strategies involved in the higher-level regulation of uncertainty in medicine (Figure 4.2). This taxonomy is based on a qualitative study my colleagues and I conducted, in which we interviewed practicing emergency medicine and internal medicine physicians about the strategies they use to manage medical uncertainty in their daily practice.[47] Participants identified a number of tertiary regulation strategies that I have categorized within a logical framework, along with additional strategies derived from both the broader

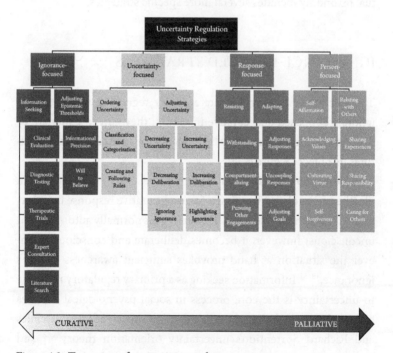

Figure 4.2 Taxonomy of uncertainty regulation strategies.

medical literature and personal observations from my past clinical experience as a general internist and palliative care physician.

The taxonomy organizes physicians' uncertainty regulation strategies according to their four primary targets: (1) ignorance, (2) uncertainty, (3) psychological responses to uncertainty, and (4) the persons (self or others) who experience uncertainty. It further categorizes these regulatory strategies according to their fundamental aims; some are curative (aimed at eliminating or reducing uncertainty), while others are palliative (aimed at ameliorating the negative psychological effects of uncertainty). Ignorance- and uncertainty-focused regulatory strategies are primarily curative, while response- and person-focused processes are primarily palliative. Within each of these broad, primary focus areas and goals, the provisional conceptual taxonomy includes several more specific strategies.

IGNORANCE-FOCUSED STRATEGIES

The first broad category of strategies for regulating uncertainty is ignorance-focused and curative in nature; they aim to eliminate or decrease medical uncertainty by reducing the ignorance that constitutes its object (Figure 4.3).

Information seeking. In medicine and every realm of human life, the predominant ignorance-focused, curative response to uncertainty is information seeking. This strategy is normally automatic and unconscious; however, it becomes deliberate and conscious whenever the situation at hand provokes sufficient awareness of one's ignorance.[48–51] Information seeking as a primary regulatory response to uncertainty is the core process in social psychological theories of knowledge, including Arie Kruglanski's theory of lay epistemics and Richard Sorrentino's uncertainty orientation theory[52,53] and theories of health communication such as Dale Brasher's uncertainty

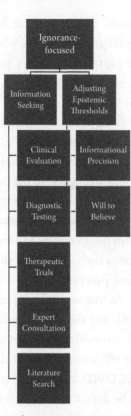

Figure 4.3 Ignorance-focused strategies.

management theory[54] and Austin Babrow's theory of problematic integration.[55,56] Information seeking is the crux of nearly all activities of clinical care, including *clinical evaluation* (enacting formal history-taking and physical examination procedures); *diagnostic testing* (conducting laboratory or imaging studies); *therapeutic trials* (enacting a course of treatment for diagnostic or prognostic purposes); *expert consultation* (accessing knowledge of other medical professionals); and *literature search* (assessing the existing corpus of medical knowledge). As sociologist Renée Fox observed, information seeking reduces not only clinicians' ignorance about the medical problem at hand but also their meta-ignorance about whether their ignorance arises from knowledge gaps that are merely personal as opposed to shared by the larger scientific community.[57]

Adjusting epistemic thresholds. Another important ignorance-focused strategy for regulating uncertainty consists of adjusting the epistemic thresholds that define the existence of knowledge or ignorance. This strategy can be accomplished by altering the precision of either one's desired knowledge or one's willingness to believe in existing evidence, which can either decrease or increase the extent of one's ignorance.

The precision of desired knowledge about any unknown outcome varies along a continuum from very low to very high. At the low end are very general questions such as whether snow is likely in winter months or whether most patients with COVID-19 pneumonia will die from their disease. At this low level of precision, questions can be definitively answered, and the corresponding level of ignorance is low. At the high end of precision, however, are very specific questions such as whether it will snow on a particular day or whether any individual patient with COVID-19 will die. At this high level of precision, questions cannot be definitively answered, and the corresponding level of ignorance is high. The precision of desired knowledge thus determines the level of ignorance, and adjusting one's *thresholds for precision* allows one to regulate one's ignorance to a more or less tolerable level. Setting the threshold of desired precision at a low level (e.g., demanding only knowledge about average outcomes of patients with COVID-19) will narrow the extent of our ignorance, while raising the threshold (e.g., demanding knowledge of the outcome of a single patient) will expand our ignorance to an unresolvable level.

But we can also regulate our ignorance is by adjusting our *will to believe*—that is, to accept versus reject—available information. Scientific researchers routinely enact this strategy in setting thresholds for hypothesis testing, which pertain to two distinct epistemic actions—accepting true propositions versus rejecting false ones. These thresholds determine the respective likelihood of two types of errors: Type I error arising from the inappropriate rejection of a null hypothesis, leading to false-positive beliefs, and Type II error arising from inappropriate acceptance of a null hypothesis, leading to false-negative beliefs. Type I error manifests excessive belief and false knowledge, whereas Type II error manifests excessive doubt and false ignorance. Adjusting the thresholds for acceptable Type I and Type II error—that is, for believing or disbelieving evidence—regulates the level of ignorance.

William James observed that exactly where one should set the epistemic thresholds for believing versus disbelieving depends on which erroneous epistemic state—false knowledge or false ignorance—has worse consequences in a given situation.[58] If false knowledge has worse consequences, then a skeptical bias toward disbelieving is more desirable; this is the general posture of scientific research. However, in other "momentous" situations, as James put it, false ignorance has worse consequences, and a bias toward believing is more desirable.[58] Such situations occur commonly in medicine. For the young mother with rapidly progressive respiratory failure from COVID-19 pneumonia, the attending physician contemplating an unproven therapy does not have the scientist's luxury of maintaining skeptical disbelief: some action must be taken or else the patient will die. The situation itself creates a powerful will to believe[58]: it pushes the physician to set his epistemic threshold at a level that favors acceptance rather than rejection of an alternative hypothesis even if it turns out to be a false-positive belief.

UNCERTAINTY-FOCUSED STRATEGIES

The second broad category of processes and strategies for regulating uncertainty is uncertainty-focused and primarily curative in nature;

strategies in this category aim at decreasing or limiting the extent not of ignorance, but of uncertainty itself (the conscious, metacognitive awareness of ignorance) (Figure 4.4).

Ordering uncertainty. A first major subcategory of uncertainty-focused regulatory strategies aims to impose order on uncertainty—a task that satisfies a basic human psychological need.[59,60] A primary cognitive process employed for this purpose is *classification*: the act of creating a "spatial, temporal, or spatio-temporal segmentation of the world," as information scientist Geoffrey Bowker and sociologist Susan Leigh Star defined it.[61] Philosopher and cognitive scientist George Lakoff used the related term *categorization* to describe this act of dividing reality into distinct entities based on their logical relationships with one another, and saw this act as fundamental to all thought, perception, action, and speech.[62] In medical practice, classification and categorization are the very foundation of diagnostic

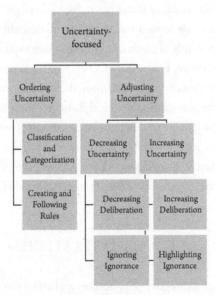

Figure 4.4 Uncertainty-focused strategies.

reasoning and medical decision-making. But they are also key strategies for regulating uncertainty. Classification and categorization impose structure and order on the otherwise unstructured, undifferentiated, "blooming, buzzing confusion"—as William James colorfully described it[63]—of human experience. Even when a diagnosis is unknown, classification and categorization reduce uncertainty by limiting diagnostic possibilities and turning them into familiar objects that are "naturalized," as Bowker and Star put it—stripped of the contingencies of their creation and taken for granted. Classification and categorization also organize clinical action, providing clinicians and patients with a feeling of security and control. They further reduce uncertainty by providing what Bowker and Star called an "information infrastructure" that serves the social, relational function of uniting individuals—in this case clinicians and patients—within common communities of practice.

Creating and following rules is another important and related strategy for ordering uncertainty. Rules guide human behavior, enabling "fast-and-frugal" decisions in the face of fundamentally limited cognitive resources[64,65] and obviating the need for experiential learning.[66] Rules also order uncertainty by promoting consistency in judgments, decisions, and outcomes.[67] In medicine, rules come in various forms, including clinical practice guidelines, standardized care pathways, and decision rules designed to promote adherence to evidence-based practices and to reduce unwarranted variation in healthcare. Less-formal versions of rules include patient treatment summaries, follow-up care plans, and even the medical record itself—all of which reinforce particular ways of interpreting and responding to clinical problems. Rules in these various forms have the common effect of reducing patients' and clinicians' uncertainty about what to expect and how to act.

Adjusting uncertainty. The other major subcategory of uncertainty-focused regulatory strategies can be either curative or palliative in intent; these strategies aim to alter the level of one's uncertainty by targeting the two psychological processes that produce it (Chapter 2): (1) active, effortful deliberation (i.e., "System 2" reasoning), and (2) perceptual awareness of novelty or discrepancy.

The first main approach, *decreasing uncertainty*, consists of two specific strategies that diminish the conscious awareness of ignorance. The first is *decreasing deliberation* by shifting from intentional, high-effort System 2 reasoning to more automatic, low-effort System 1 reasoning. The second strategy is *ignoring ignorance*—that is, decreasing the conscious perception of ignorance by diverting attention away from its sources. Both strategies may be enacted either unintentionally as a result of mental fatigue, distraction, or competing attentional demands or intentionally as a conscious, active effort to maintain psychological well-being. In any case, the finite cognitive capacity of the human mind and the aversive nature of uncertainty require us at some point to let go of our ignorance and our efforts to resolve it. This was the task advocated in the ancient Greek philosophy of skepticism, which idealized the "suspension of judgment" as a way of achieving *ataraxia*, or "freedom from disturbance or calmness of soul."[68–71]

The converse approach consists of *increasing uncertainty* through two more specific strategies. The first is *increasing deliberation* by shifting from System 1 to System 2 reasoning. This is a primary goal of the idealized process of shared decision-making (SDM), which aims to help clinicians and patients engage in "collaborative deliberation" about the benefits, harms, and uncertainties of preference-sensitive medical interventions for which there is clinical equipoise regarding their net value.[72] The ultimate aim is not to decrease but to increase uncertainty and to help patients make decisions in spite of it. The second strategy is *highlighting ignorance*—that is, increasing the conscious perception of ignorance by focusing attention on its sources. These include the indeterminacy and indeterminability of health outcomes, which are manifest, respectively, by probability and ambiguity in existing information (Chapter 3). SDM conversations often highlight the indeterminacy and indeterminability of health outcomes in order to help patients understand the level of scientific uncertainty about a given medical intervention.[73]

But the act of highlighting these sources of ignorance is equally important in coping efforts of patients with serious life-limiting illnesses such as cancer. For such patients, prognostic uncertainty is a primary source not of fear but of hope because it leaves open the possibility of a good outcome.[74-77] Consequently, many patients with life-limiting illness actively strive not to decrease but to increase prognostic uncertainty—to construct and maintain it through various strategies. These include acknowledging the fundamental limitations of prognostic knowledge (e.g., by highlighting the indeterminacy of prognosis and the ambiguity of prognostic information), relinquishing the pursuit of prognostic knowledge, and embracing ignorance (e.g., by avoiding prognostic information altogether). My own research has shown that the active, intentional highlighting of ignorance arising from indeterminacy and indeterminability represents a key coping strategy that enables patients with advanced cancer to achieve an adaptive, dynamic balance between fear and hope.[78] For these patients, prognostic uncertainty is not an aversive but an attractive state that they strive to maintain.

RESPONSE-FOCUSED STRATEGIES

The next broad category of regulatory processes and strategies focuses not on uncertainty itself, but on people's primary psychological responses to it (Figure 4.5). Strategies in this category are primarily palliative rather than curative in nature: they aim to ameliorate the

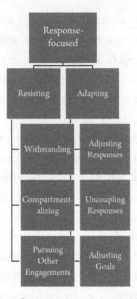

Figure 4.5 Response-focused strategies.

various negative cognitive, emotional, and behavioral responses that comprise the syndromes of risk, ambiguity, and complexity aversion.

Resisting. One major subcategory of response-focused regulatory strategies aims at resisting negative psychological effects of uncertainty. The first of these strategies, *withstanding,* refers to somehow enduring these effects and maintaining well-being in the face of adversity. It manifests a fundamental human capacity that psychologists and philosophers since the time of the ancient Greek Stoics have described using terms such as *fortitude* and *resilience.*[79–81] *Compartmentalizing* is a strategy that also aims at resisting the negative effects of uncertainty, but in an avoidant fashion that restricts attention to one's these effects—sequestering them from awareness. In psychological theories of coping, these strategies would be classified as "avoidant coping" processes that ultimately aim to ignore or avoid the existence of the problem at hand, and to dissociate oneself from it.[82-84] This strategy can be enacted unintentionally through "denial" and intentionally through strategies such as distraction and relaxation.[12,83-85] *Pursuing other engagements* is a final response-resisting strategy involving participation in activities that focus one's attention beyond medical uncertainty and its aversive effects. For physicians and other health professionals, this strategy can involve a variety of professional and leisure pursuits outside of medicine, including nonclinical professional activities (e.g., research, teaching, administration) and personal activities (e.g., hobbies, caring for one's family). The pursuit of such engagements can be an essential strategy for coping with uncertainty and averting professional burnout.

Adapting. Another important subcategory of response-focused regulatory strategies aims not at resisting but at altering one's aversive responses to uncertainty. *Adjusting responses* entails directly modifying them in various ways, including reframing, reevaluating, and adopting new cognitive perspectives or behavioral approaches to uncertainty. Such strategies have been incorporated in cognitive behavioral therapy interventions used to treat pathological anxiety disorders,[83-87] which some clinical psychologists attribute to intolerance of uncertainty.[12,88,89] A related strategy, *uncoupling responses*, involves dissociating particular cognitive, emotional, and behavioral responses to uncertainty from one another. In most circumstances, these responses co-occur in the same psychologically consistent combinations that comprise the syndromes of risk, ambiguity, and complexity aversion (i.e., heightened perceptions of vulnerability, fear, and decision avoidance). An important adaptive response to uncertainty, however, involves uncoupling and recombining these responses in ways that may be psychologically inconsistent but adaptive. Many difficult medical situations require patients and clinicians to make decisions in spite of how vulnerable or fearful their uncertainty makes them feel. The patient and physician contemplating an unproven, both potentially beneficial and harmful therapy for worsening COVID-19 pneumonia (e.g., high-dose steroids) must eventually make a decision, no matter how risky it may feel. Similarly, this and many other serious life-limiting illnesses require both patients and clinicians to maintain dissonant combinations of hope and fear, optimism and pessimism, in the face of prognostic uncertainty. For physicians, uncoupling is also manifest in what Renée Fox called the posture of "detached concern," which enables them to be at once empathic and impersonal in their approach to their patients—to maintain sufficient psychological distance to avoid being consumed by the emotional distress of others and to exercise sound clinical judgment.[90]

Adjusting goals is a final important response-focused strategy for regulating uncertainty. Social psychologists Charles Carver and Michael Scheier have highlighted the central role of this strategy in the self-regulation of behavior.[91,92] In their view, goals are mental representations of desired states of being and occupy a hierarchy ranging from higher-level, moral goals to lower-level, instrumental goals. People constantly monitor their goals and make adjustments whenever they are not achieved—including letting go of some goals and replacing them with others. Uncertainty is one of the most important causes of such goal adjustments, as the COVID-19 pandemic has demonstrated: uncertainty about the course and severity of the pandemic has prompted a massive shift in both individual and societal goals at various levels. At the highest moral level, goals of physical well-being and the collective good have taken precedence over goals of short-term economic well-being and personal freedom, while at lower instrumental levels, tasks such as the maintenance of social distancing and lockdowns have become key goals. As an uncertainty regulation strategy, goal adjustment can also involve relinquishing or deemphasizing goals whose achievement is more uncertain, and focusing on goals whose achievement is more certain. Whether the goal of survival will be achieved for the young mother with severe

COVID-19 pneumonia, for example, is unknowable; one way for her care team to regulate their uncertainty about this goal is not to abandon its pursuit, but to focus on more certainly attainable goals such the emotional and spiritual well-being of the patient and her family. Such goal adjustments can have other psychological and moral benefits; however, the point here is that they also represent a primary strategy for regulating and adapting to uncertainty.

An equally important type of goal adjustment pertains to epistemic goals—that is, to the degree of certainty or knowledge that one pursues and expects. In many circumstances in medicine, ignorance is irreducible, and a high degree of certainty is simply impossible. In such situations, clinicians and patients must relax their epistemic goals and expectations; they must adopt mature epistemic beliefs that affirm the irreducibility of ignorance and the unattainability of absolute certainty. They must relinquish the quest for certainty in favor of more attainable goals.

PERSON-FOCUSED STRATEGIES

The final broad category of strategies for regulating uncertainty focuses not on uncertainty, ignorance, or individuals' negative psychological responses to uncertainty, but on the individuals themselves (self or others) who experience uncertainty. These person-focused strategies for regulating uncertainty are exclusively palliative in nature; they aim at ameliorating uncertainty's psychologically aversive effects (Figure 4.6).

Self-affirmation. A major subcategory of person-focused regulatory strategies aims at helping clinicians and patients to affirm themselves. Self-affirmation, as originally described by social psychologist Claude Steele, signifies a process by which one protects and maintains self-integrity—that is, the concept of oneself as a

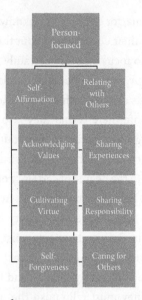

Figure 4.6 Person-focused strategies.

good person—by reflecting on one's most fundamental values and beliefs.[93–95] A large body of empirical research has demonstrated how self-affirmation helps people cope with new information or experiences that threaten self-integrity, and emerging evidence also suggests that self-affirmation also reduces maladaptive responses to uncertainties related to people's health.[94,96]

Self-affirmation can be accomplished through various strategies. *Acknowledging personal values* is the primary strategy examined in past empirical research on self-affirmation. It is also a core component of the idealized process of SDM—suggesting that SDM may serve a dual function of enabling patients not only to make value-concordant choices but to cope with the uncertainty generated by these choices. *Cultivating virtue* is a closely related task that goes beyond simply acknowledging key personal values to actualizing them through one's behaviors. The critical care physician caring for her COVID-19 patient may actualize values of diligence, thoroughness, and devotion to her patient's welfare, for example, by continually reevaluating her patient and pursuing an exhaustive diagnostic workup in an effort to "leave no stone unturned." Cultivating such virtues protects the physician against the threat of uncertainty by preserving her sense of self-integrity and directing her attention toward higher-level ideals that give meaning to her actions—and away from her uncertainty.

Self-forgiveness is a final self-affirmation strategy of great importance to clinicians as well as patients. For physicians, much of the aversiveness of medical uncertainty originates from the threat of being wrong—of making mistakes with dire consequences for patients. To handle this threat in an adaptive manner, physicians must be able to have mercy on themselves—to let go of self-blame and the demand for self-perfection when reality falls short of expectations. Many system and individual-level factors mitigate against this capacity, however, including professional values and norms, the threat of malpractice litigation, and personality differences, such as the "fear of invalidity," among physicians and patients.[60] These and other factors influence every individual's capacity to respond adaptively to undesired outcomes, and to accept themselves in spite of these outcomes.

Relating with others. The other major subcategory of person-focused uncertainty regulatory strategies consists of activities directed not inwardly at one's own self, but outwardly toward other human beings and one's interpersonal interactions with them. Central to these activities is the act of *sharing experiences.* This process serves the function of creating what psychologists Maya Rossignac-Milon and E. Tory Higgins have called a "generalized shared reality": a common worldview, comprising beliefs, feelings, and concerns, which provides a sense of order.[97-100] The uncertainty-regulating effect of this sharing process, however, is not just informational but also emotional and relational. Rossignac-Milon and Higgins have argued that "jointly satisfying epistemic needs—making sense of the world together—bonds partners at various relationship phases"[101]; it establishes a perceived commonality of inner states that itself has an important uncertainty-regulating effect. As they have put it vividly, "humans are truth-cartographers searching for epistemic companions with whom to map out the bounds of reality. Finding another person with whom one can intimately understand and makes sense of the world fosters a sense of epistemic glue."[101] The very act of sharing experiences—no matter what specific information might be exchanged in the process—protects people against a sense of existential isolation,[102] increases subjective well-being,[98,103] and thus helps people cope with uncertainty. In the face of uncertainty about what the future holds, sharing experiences allows the critically ill mother with COVID-19 and members of her medical team to be present with one another as epistemic companions. Simply facing uncertainty together—rather than alone—may be one of the most powerful ways for both parties to regulate their responses to it.

Sharing responsibility, the next relational strategy, focuses on distributing the moral and practical burdens of managing uncertainty, making it easier for any one person to bear. Examples of this strategy include SDM as well as interprofessional team care, which aims to foster collaboration and distribute decision-making responsibility among physicians, patients, and other health professionals. These strategies are justified by multiple values and goals: respect for patient autonomy, healthcare quality and safety, patient and provider satisfaction. By distributing responsibility for managing uncertainty, these endeavors also enable individuals to regulate their responses to it.

The final, arguably most important relational strategy for regulating uncertainty is *caring for others*—an act that goes beyond simply sharing experiences or responsibility to actively helping another person. Caring is the ultimate goal of medicine as an institution; however, Arthur Kleinman recognized that it serves deeper ends.

He argued that the very act of caring for a fellow human being is the most profound of all existential experiences and imperatives.[104] In actualizing a commitment to doing good for others, caring not only holds society together but also enables us to transcend our uncertainty: to move forward regardless of our ignorance about what lies ahead. Through caring we affirm our shared needs and condition as human beings: "By giving care, we recognize that we, too, need to be cared for," Kleinman observed. As a participatory affirmation of our shared existential state, caring empowers us to face the threat of the unknown.

THE TERTIARY REGULATION OF UNCERTAINTY

I have developed a conceptual framework that describes the natural history of uncertainty in terms of two main sets of psychological responses: (1) primary, consisting of aversive cognitive, emotional, and behavioral responses to risk, ambiguity, and complexity, and (2) secondary, consisting of compensatory strategies for regulating these primary aversive responses. The framework further categorizes these secondary regulatory strategies according to their substantive focus (ignorance-focused, uncertainty-focused, response-focused, and person-focused) and fundamental nature (curative vs. palliative). This framework is by no means definitive or complete; more work is needed to capture the full range of secondary uncertainty regulation strategies and their relationships with one another. In the meantime, however, the framework provides an initial way for clinicians and patients to take stock of these strategies and to attain some level of tertiary metacognitive control over them.

The problem, however, is that we do not yet know what uncertainty regulation strategies or combinations of strategies are most effective, in which circumstances, and why. Much more empirical research is needed to answer these questions; however, the conceptual framework can be useful in this effort as well. It can enable researchers to measure and assess the effectiveness of different strategies for regulating uncertainty and to develop causal theories that explain why clinicians and patients employ different strategies and what effects these strategies have.[84–87] In her influential uncertainty in illness theory, for example, nursing researcher and uncertainty scholar Merle Mishel posited that initial positive and negative appraisals of uncertainty promote problem-focused versus emotion-focused coping strategies.[105,106] The current conceptual framework suggests the need to extend this theory by identifying additional coping strategies that focus on a variety of other important targets: ignorance, uncertainty itself, one's psychological responses to uncertainty, oneself and others. Some strategies are curative, while others are palliative in intent. Some aim to alter uncertainty itself, while others aim to alter one's responses to it. Some involve approaching uncertainty, while others involve avoiding it. By focusing attention on these other strategies and the distinctions between them, the current framework can guide future work to better understand how clinicians and patients regulate medical uncertainty.

The ultimate goal of this framework, however, is practical: to improve the management of uncertainty in medicine. The framework can promote this goal by enabling clinicians and patients to rise above their own regulatory responses to uncertainty and to achieve greater tertiary control over them. Yet the framework does not provide guidance on what specific strategies an individual clinician or patient ought to implement in order to manage the variety of uncertainties that arise in medicine. This is not a descriptive question about the natural history of uncertainty, but a normative question about the goals of uncertainty management and the best approach to the task. I next attempt to address this difficult question and to derive a practically useful normative framework for the management of uncertainty in medicine.

Chapter 5

The Management of Uncertainty

I make no pretense of omniscience. Decisions about diagnosis and treatment are complex. There are dark corners to every clinical situation. Knowledge in medicine is imperfect. No diagnostic test is flawless. No drug is without side effects, expected or idiosyncratic. No prognosis is fully predictable. Still, there are important landmarks that help doctor and patient successfully navigate this uncertain terrain.

—Jerome Groopman[1]

Managing uncertainty is a metacognitive endeavor that requires clinicians and patients to reflect on their uncertainties and their actual and potential responses to it and to enact responses that are most appropriate to the situation at hand. The challenge of this endeavor, however, is that the appropriateness of different responses to uncertainty is a normative question. It depends on what the ultimate goals of managing medical uncertainty ought to be, and this question has yet to be answered. There are multiple potential goals, but to my knowledge there have been no previous attempts to articulate and prioritize them. Furthermore, we lack a coherent overarching strategy for evaluating and managing medical uncertainty in a systematic, goal-directed manner.

In this chapter, I venture into uncertain terrain by identifying a provisional set of normative goals for the management of uncertainty in medicine and discuss their rationale. I then propose an overarching practical framework that operationalizes uncertainty management in

Uncertainty in Medicine. Paul K.J. Han, Oxford University Press. © Oxford University Press 2021.
DOI: 10.1093/oso/9780190270582.003.0005

terms of the same key tasks that comprise the clinical management of all medical problems: establishing a diagnosis, assessing prognosis, clarifying goals, and determining treatment. I conclude by illustrating the potential usefulness of the framework in helping clinicians and patients evaluate and manage medical uncertainty in a more intentional, systematic, goal-directed manner.

GOALS OF UNCERTAINTY MANAGEMENT

The goals of managing uncertainty in medicine can be classified within a hierarchy according to their nature and level of abstraction. At the primary, concrete level are proximate goals, which are practical in nature and focus on the immediate outcomes of different uncertainty management strategies; in the framework of Carver and Scheier, these represent "do goals."[2,3] At the higher, abstract level are ultimate goals, which are moral in nature and focus on the superordinate values and principles that define an ideal human existence; these represent "be goals."

Proximate goals: cure and palliation. The primary lower-level, concrete, proximate goals of managing uncertainty parallel the goals of managing most medical problems and consist of cure and palliation. Like the illnesses that represent the primary focus of medical care, uncertainty is generally an aversive condition that both clinicians and patients strive to either eliminate or endure. The many strategies that both parties use to regulate uncertainty thus aim to achieve at least one of these two goals (Chapter 4). Ignorance-focused strategies (seeking information, adjusting epistemic thresholds) and uncertainty-focused strategies (ordering uncertainty, disengaging from uncertainty) are primarily curative; they aim to eliminate or reduce uncertainty by decreasing either ignorance itself or the conscious awareness of it. Response-focused strategies (resisting uncertainty, adapting to uncertainty) and person-focused strategies (self-affirmation, relating with others), on the other hand, are primarily palliative; they aim to ameliorate the negative psychological effects of uncertainty.

These proximate goals of cure and palliation are not mutually exclusive, however; some uncertainty regulation strategies—uncertainty-focused and response-focused strategies in particular—aim at both reducing uncertainty and ameliorating negative responses to it. As for most medical illnesses, furthermore, complete "cure" of the "illness" of uncertainty is simply impossible due to the ineradicable nature of many of the root causes of medical ignorance (Chapter 3). Nevertheless, the concepts of cure and palliation capture key functions that are served by clinicians' and patients' efforts to manage medical uncertainty. Identifying cure and palliation as normative goals simply makes these functions explicit, so that clinicians and patients can manage uncertainty in a more intentional, goal-directed manner.

Ultimate goals: uncertainty tolerance. But these proximate goals alone are not sufficient to guide the management of medical uncertainty. Simply deciding whether the goals of any given uncertainty management strategy should be curative or palliative does not answer the question of the strategy's appropriateness. A primary reason is that uncertainty, unlike most medical conditions that clinicians and patients manage, has not only negative but also positive psychological effects. Positive cognitive effects include perceptions of hope and confidence; positive emotional effects include feelings of curiosity and excitement; positive behavioral effects include engagement and motivation to act. For the clinically deteriorating patient receiving a novel, unproven therapy for severe COVID-19 pneumonia, for example, prognostic and therapeutic uncertainty can be a source of not only despair, fear, and resignation, but also hope, engagement, and commitment. The dual, positive-and-negative nature of these and other medical uncertainties makes it difficult to determine whether they should be cured or palliated.

Compounding this difficulty, the effects of uncertainty vary depending on the individual. A large body of empirical research, dating back to the 1949 work of psychologist Else Frenkel-Brunswik,[4] has shown that individuals differ in their *uncertainty tolerance* (UT).[5-7] Some individuals, Frenkel-Brunswik observed, are less capable than others of "seeing things in two or more different ways" and demonstrate a "reluctance to think in terms of probabilities and a preference to escape into whatever seems definite and therefore safe."[4] Since then, several researchers have refined the concept of UT and measured its extent and relationship to various psychological outcomes.[5] Psychologist Nicholas Carleton, who developed one of the most widely used measures of UT, defined intolerance of uncertainty as "an individual's dispositional incapacity to endure the aversive response triggered by the perceived absence of salient, key, or sufficient information, and sustained by the associated perception of uncertainty."[7] Empirical studies have demonstrated that UT varies widely and is associated with various personality traits and psychological outcomes.[5] In particular, lower UT (greater intolerance of uncertainty) is associated with worry and anxiety[8-10] and is thought to play a causal role in the pathogenesis of generalized anxiety disorder, panic disorder, social anxiety disorder, phobias, obsessive-compulsive disorder, and depression.[11-13] Individual differences in UT and its psychological effects adds to the difficulty of determining whether any given medical uncertainty should be cured or palliated for any given individual or situation.

Determining the appropriate management of uncertainty is thus a complex task that requires more than deciding whether uncertainty should be cured or palliated, reduced or endured. It requires justifying this decision with reference to higher-level, moral goals—that is, the ultimate be goals that specify how people ought to live with uncertainty. The question is, what should these ultimate moral goals be? One possibility, implied in traditional conceptualizations of UT, is greater net "positivity" in the sum total of an individual's psychological responses to uncertainty. Measures of individual differences in UT, for example, generally assess the extent to which individuals exhibit various negative, aversive psychological responses to uncertainty and simply aggregate these responses to produce a summary score. Scores that are more negative indicate lower UT, while scores that are more positive indicate higher UT.

For several reasons, however, UT in this sense—of more positively valenced psychological responses to uncertainty—is not an appropriate moral goal for uncertainty management. To treat it as such would be to regard psychologically negative responses as exclusively maladaptive and morally undesirable, and positive ones as exclusively adaptive and desirable. Yet there is no straightforward 1:1 correspondence between the psychological and moral valence of individuals' responses to uncertainty; moral valence depends on the individual and circumstance. For some individuals and circumstances, psychologically "negative" perceptions of vulnerability, feelings of fear, and decision avoidance—the hallmarks of ambiguity aversion—can be morally "positive" in promoting appropriate caution in the face of uncertainty. They can prompt the desperate patient contemplating an unproven and potentially dangerous medical intervention to stop, think, and seek essential information before taking action. Conversely, psychologically positive responses such as confidence and hope can be morally negative in leading the patient to make a reckless decision.

Furthermore, people's varied positive and negative cognitive, emotional, and behavioral responses to uncertainty do not—and should not—always move in lockstep with one another. Both clinicians and patients must often uncouple and compartmentalize particular responses from one another (Chapter 4); for example, many medical circumstances demand courageous and decisive action in spite of ongoing doubt and fear. Other circumstances require clinicians and patients to intentionally combine various uncertainty regulation strategies in logically inconsistent—but psychologically adaptive—ways. Examples include the posture of "detached concern"[14,15] that clinicians often assume when caring for seriously ill patients, and the simultaneous maintenance of optimism and pessimism that seriously ill patients strive for in "hoping for the best while preparing for the worst."[16] Tolerating uncertainty often requires dissonant combinations of responses such as these.

For all of these reasons, the ultimate moral goal of uncertainty management cannot consist simply of greater net positivity in the psychological valence of individuals' responses to uncertainty, or of any particular combination of negative or positive cognitive, emotional, or behavioral responses. There is no single, universal, "right" answer to the question of how to manage uncertainty in medicine or any realm of human life: it all depends on the individual, the uncertainty, and the situation. This means that the ultimate moral goal of uncertainty management must consist of UT in a broader sense: *the capacity to achieve an optimal, adaptive balance of responses to uncertainty.* This balance is a dynamic state of equilibrium that encompasses the totality of psychological responses to uncertainty—both negative and positive in valence, and cognitive, emotional, and behavioral in nature. The net balance of responses will sometimes be more psychologicaclly negative and other times more positive. Sometimes the particular combination of responses will be logically consistent; other times it will be inconsistent. What determines the moral appropriateness of any particular set of responses is not its psychological positivity or logical consistency, but the extent to which it enables individuals to adapt to the uncertainties they experience. This depends, in turn, on each individual's own needs, values, and goals, as well as the particulars of the situation. UT in this higher-level, moral sense allows these individual factors to be accounted for. It is the adaptive capacity that empowers individuals to rise above and manage their own responses to their own unique uncertainties in a way that works best for them.

Arthur Kleinman closed his book *What Really Matters* with a metaphor that beautifully illustrates the meaning of UT in this higher-level, moral sense. Reflecting on Picasso's abstract painting *The Head of a Medical Student* (Figure 5.1)—which depicts a face with one eye open, the other eye closed—Kleinman offered the following interpretation:

> *Medical students learn to open one eye to the pain and suffering of patients and the world, but also to close the other eye—to protect their own vulnerability to pain and suffering, to protect their belief that they can do good and change the world for the better, to protect their own self-interests such as career building and economic gain. I would generalize the provocative poignancy of this picture to how we live our lives. One of our eyes is open to the dangers of the world and the uncertainty of our human condition; the other is closed, so that we do not see or feel these things, so that we can get on with our lives. But perhaps one eye is closed so that we can see, feel and do something of value. One eye, perhaps, sees the possibilities and hopefulness of who we are and where we are headed, while the other is shut tight with fear over the storms and precipices that lie ahead.*[17]

This metaphor applies not only to medical students but also to clinicians, patients, and all of us as human beings experiencing the manifold uncertainties of medicine and human life. At any given moment, we respond to these uncertainties by enacting opposing regulatory strategies focused on different targets: our ignorance, our uncertainty, our responses to uncertainty, our selves. We either seek information to resolve our ignorance or adjust our epistemic expectations

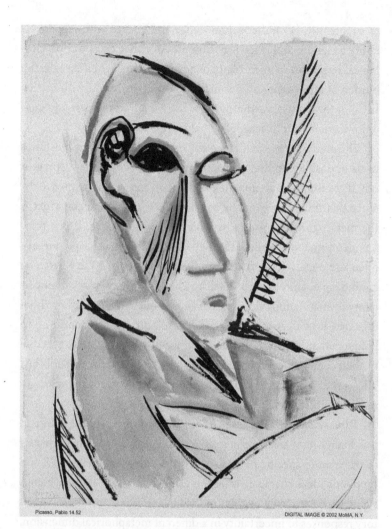

Figure 5.1   *Head of a Medical Student* (Pablo Picasso, 1907). *Source:* © *2021 Estate of Pablo Picasso/Artists Rights Society (ARS), New York.*

to suppress it. We either acknowledge and engage with our uncertainty or ignore and disengage from it. We either resist our psychological responses to uncertainty or adapt to them. We either take the burden of uncertainty on our own shoulders or share it with others. In all of these ways, furthermore, we strive either to resist and cure our uncertainty or to accept and palliate it.

The metaphor of simultaneously open and closed eyes illustrates these opposing impulses and actions and shows how they represent not dichotomies but dualities—essential aspects of human existence that must somehow be balanced. UT as a moral construct is the metacognitive capacity to achieve these functions. It is a transcendent, metauncertain, "third-eye" awareness that keeps one eye open and one eye closed and handles the binocular rivalry between conflicting cognitive, emotional, and behavioral responses to uncertainty by maintaining them, rather than abolishing or blending them together. It is a capacity to take on contradiction and tension—to hold together disparate elements that would normally split apart due to their logical incoherence or their psychological incompatibility. This is the core meaning of UT as a normative goal for the management of uncertainty.

Dimensions of tolerance: humility, flexibility, courage. But in this higher-level sense of metacognitive balance, UT itself consists of three more specific be goals—moral virtues that enable UT and represent ideal character traits or dispositions that human beings aspire to. Each virtue enables individuals to transcend their regulatory responses to uncertainty in a different metaphorical dimension, and thus represents a distinct integral component of UT.

The first virtue, *humility*, enables transcendence in a vertical dimension—allowing individuals to rise above both their uncertainty and their responses to uncertainty in the first place, and to achieve the tertiary metacognitive consciousness needed to manage them. Humility is a complex concept that philosophers and psychologists have conceived in various ways.[18,19] A particularly useful construct for the current analysis is *intellectual humility*—defined by philosopher Dennis Whitcomb as a disposition to be aware of one's limitations in knowledge[20] and by philosopher Alan Hazlett as "a disposition not to adopt epistemically improper higher-order epistemic attitudes, and to adopt (in the right way, in the right situations) epistemically proper higher-order epistemic attitudes."[21] At its core, the concept of intellectual humility represents a particular epistemic disposition— an orientation of openness toward acknowledging ignorance and both achieving and maintaining uncertainty.[22-24] Humility in this sense is a necessary precondition for uncertainty and all subsequent efforts to manage it; without humility we could not rise above and become aware of our ignorance, let alone regulate our responses to it. Humility orients us vertically: toward making the quantum leap from ignorance to uncertainty and ultimately from uncertainty to metauncertainty—the higher-level metacognitive state that makes it possible to balance and integrate our multiple different responses to uncertainty. Humility is thus an integral component of UT.

The second virtue, *flexibility*, enables transcendence in a horizontal dimension—allowing individuals to move across their diverse, conflicting psychological responses to uncertainty and to adjust their mix—that is, to find an adaptive balance of responses in a given situation. Like humility, flexibility has been conceptualized in multiple ways; however, one construct, *psychological flexibility* (PF), is particularly useful for our purposes. Psychologist Stephen Hayes has defined PF as "the ability to contact the present moment more fully as a conscious human being, and to change or persist in behavior when doing so serves valued ends."[25] Psychologists Todd Kashdan and Jonathan Rottenberg have defined PF more specifically as the "ability to modify responses to best match the situation," which serves multiple self-regulatory functions, including to "recognize and adapt to various situational demands; shift mindsets or behavioral repertoires when these strategies compromise personal or social functioning; maintain balance among important life domains; and be aware, open, and committed to behaviors that are congruent with deeply held values."[26] At its core, the concept of PF represents a cognitive capacity to shift attention when needed, an emotional capacity to apply "different types of emotional expression as the situation warrants," and a behavioral capacity "to find alternative routes toward desired ends"—all of which ultimately enable us to adapt to an "uncertain, unpredictable world" in which "novelty and change are the norm rather than the exception."[26] Flexibility orients us horizontally: toward balancing our many opposing, negative versus positive psychological responses to uncertainty—uncoupling and recombining them in adaptive ways. Flexibility is thus an integral component of UT.

The third virtue, *courage*, enables transcendence in a forward dimension—allowing individuals to move ahead from the known present to the unknown future, in spite of their uncertainty and their conflicting responses to it, in order to get on with their lives. Like humility and flexibility, courage has been defined in numerous ways. Psychologist Stanley Rachman has defined courage as "persistence in dealing with a dangerous situation despite subjective and physical signs of fear,"[27] while Cooper Woodard and Cynthia Pury has defined it as "the voluntary willingness to act, with or without varying levels of fear, in response to a threat to achieve an important, perhaps moral, outcome or goal."[28] At its core, the concept of courage represents a capacity to resist fear and take action to achieve some particular goal; however, courage has not only psychological but also existential connotations. Existentialist theologian Paul Tillich viewed courage as the capacity to resist the profound despair caused by the "threat of nonbeing"—the recognition of the finite nature of one's existence.[29] For Tillich, courage meant a broader, overarching "courage to be"—a transcendent "self-affirmation of being in spite of the fact of nonbeing"[29]—that enables individuals to accept their many fatal flaws (biological, moral, and spiritual) that stem from human finitude, and to go on living in spite of them. In a similar vein, psychologist Rollo May defined courage as "the capacity to meet the anxiety which arises as one achieves freedom": to overcome the "fear of moving ahead" and to engage in "acting, loving, thinking, creating, even though one knows he does not have the final answers, and he may well be wrong."[30] Courage in this larger, existential sense ultimately orients us forward: toward taking action and leaping ahead into the unknown and affirming our own existence in spite of all that threatens it. Courage thus represents the final, most decisive component of UT.

MANAGING UNCERTAINTY IN MEDICINE: AN INTEGRATIVE FRAMEWORK

I have identified a set of normative goals for uncertainty management, which I have classified within a two-level hierarchy according to their nature and level of abstraction. At the lower, concrete, proximate level are the practical goals of *cure* and *palliation* (do goals). At the higher, abstract, ultimate level is the overarching moral goal of *tolerance* in the broad sense of the transcendent, metacognitive, third-eye capacity to achieve an optimal, adaptive, dynamic balance of responses to uncertainty. The three moral virtues—*humility*, *flexibility*, and *courage*—that are integral components of UT (be goals) also reside at this higher, ultimate level. Together, these proximate and ultimate goals represent guiding principles for efforts to manage uncertainty in medicine.

Before they can serve this function, however, these normative goals must somehow be integrated within uncertainty management efforts. What clinicians and patients need is a coherent, overarching strategy that can enable them to evaluate and manage their uncertainties in both a goal-directed and systematic manner. Toward this end, I now propose a provisional framework that operationalizes uncertainty management in terms of the same prototypical tasks that constitute the management of all important medical problems: (1) establishing a diagnosis, (2) assessing prognosis, (3) clarifying goals, and (4) determining treatment. These tasks aim to answer key questions about the nature, etiology, anatomy, and natural history of the uncertainties experienced by clinicians or patients, as well as the goals of managing these uncertainties.

Figure 5.2 provides a visual representation of this integrative framework for uncertainty management. The first task, *establishing the diagnosis*, addresses key questions about the nature and etiology of one's uncertainty, focusing on the three fundamental dimensions of all uncertainties (source, issue, and locus): *(1) What are the sources, or root causes, of this uncertainty? (2) What substantive issues are the objects of this uncertainty? (3) In whose minds does this uncertainty exist, and to what extent is it shared among different individuals?* The answers to these questions provide an anatomical shape and form to uncertainty, enabling clinicians and patients to stand apart from it, determine its importance, and manage it systematically.

The next task, *assessing prognosis*, addresses another key question about the anticipated outcomes of managing the uncertainty at hand: *To what extent is this uncertainty reducible or irreducible?* The answer to this question helps set appropriate expectations for efforts to manage these uncertainties and one's psychological responses to them. It helps clarify the extent to which these efforts should be directed more toward curative strategies (aimed at reducing either ignorance or uncertainty), as opposed to palliative strategies (aimed at the minimization of suffering and the maximization of benefits associated with uncertainty).

The next task, *clarifying goals*, addresses the pivotal question: *What are the objectives of managing a given uncertainty?* The first

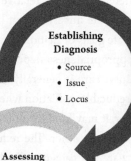

Establishing Diagnosis
- Source
- Issue
- Locus

Assessing Prognosis
- Reducible
- Irreducible

Determining Treatment
- Ignorance-focused
- Uncertainty-focused
- Response-focused
- Person-focused

Clarifying Goals
- Cure
- Palliation
- Tolerance
  - Humility
  - Flexibility
  - Courage

Figure 5.2 Integrative framework of uncertainty management.

task involves determining the relative appropriateness of different goals in managing the uncertainty at hand. Cure and palliation are primary proximate goals of all individual management strategies, and their relative appropriateness depends primarily on the prognosis of the uncertainty: cure is generally the appropriate goal when the uncertainty is reducible, palliation when it is irreducible. For several reasons, however, it may be difficult for clinicians or patients to prioritize one goal or the other. The reducibility and irreducibility of any uncertainty are not categorically distinct, either/or characteristics, but continuous qualities that vary along a continuum. Whether a given uncertainty is sufficiently reducible or irreducible to warrant curative versus palliative treatment, therefore, is a matter of judgment. Furthermore, although some uncertainties might be reducible in theory, the appropriate management strategy might be palliative rather than curative; it depends on the individual and situation. Finally, for any given uncertainty the goals of managing uncertainty may be ambiguous or mixed; both cure and palliation may be appropriate, and a combination of different management strategies may thus be indicated.

This is where tolerance, the third, higher-level goal, comes into play. When uncertainties are not clearly reducible or irreducible or when the goals of management are ambiguous or mixed, clinicians and patients need to accept this ambiguity and strike an appropriate balance between multiple goals and management strategies. Tolerance becomes the overarching goal, and humility, flexibility, and courage—the three moral virtues that make up tolerance—become key instrumental goals that may each serve particularly important functions, depending on the situation. Humility, for example, may be especially important when clinicians and patients first confront a medical problem and need to rise above their uncertainty and assess its sources, issues, locus, and effects.[31] Flexibility and courage may be more important as uncertainties and decision options multiply, requiring clinicians and patients to creatively integrate different potential responses to uncertainty and to eventually move forward in spite of it.

The final task and ultimate goal of managing medical uncertainty, *determining treatment*, answers the pragmatic question, *How should this uncertainty be managed?* Answering this question requires synthesizing insights from all of the preceding tasks to select an appropriate management strategy from the full array of potential ignorance-, uncertainty-, response-, and person-focused responses, both curative and palliative (Chapter 4). Determining which of these strategies is appropriate for any given uncertainty in any given situation depends on the diagnosis and prognosis of the uncertainty and the proximate and ultimate goals of managing it. The task of determining treatment actualizes UT. It requires and manifests the higher-level metacognitive capacity—the third-eye state of metauncertainty—to regulate one's own uncertainty and one's primary and secondary responses to it. It enables clinicians and patients to select tertiary management strategies that achieve an optimal balance between differing responses, given the particulars of the situation.

The interlocking circles in Figure 5.2 represent the interdependent, mutually reinforcing nature of each of these management tasks; they build on one another and culminate in a treatment determination that integrates all of the information gained through the other tasks. This determination is never definitive, however, given that medical uncertainty and its many psychological effects constantly evolve in response to—and often in spite of—efforts to manage them. The component processes of uncertainty management depicted in Figure 5.2 are thus provisional and bidirectional. They are iteratively updated in response to changes in either one's uncertainties or their effects, which may require revising one's diagnostic, prognostic assessments or management goals. Uncertainty management, in other words, is a continuously evolving process.

A FRAMEWORK-GUIDED APPROACH TO UNCERTAINTY MANAGEMENT: CASE STUDY

This integrative framework is a normative rather than a descriptive model; it specifies how clinicians and patients ideally should manage uncertainty, not how they actually do manage it. It outlines a rational approach consisting of a few well-defined, stepwise tasks that mirror the management of all medical problems. The framework does not, however, designate any particular uncertainty management strategy as rational or not, nor does it provide definitive answers to the question of what strategies are appropriate in any given situation. Rather, it assumes that the appropriate uncertainty management strategy depends on the personal values, preferences, and needs of individual clinicians and patients, as well as the particulars of the situation. Just as there is no one right medical decision when scientific evidence is lacking or the benefits and harms of medical intervention are unclear, there is no one right way of managing uncertainty. Like the idealized model of shared decision-making in medicine, therefore, this framework prescribes not an outcome but a process, not a definitive answer but a provisional approach to an answer. It supports the autonomy of individual clinicians and patients to determine for themselves how uncertainty ought to be managed.

The inability of this framework to prescribe single right answers means that it will not necessarily make the management of uncertainty any easier. However, I believe it can at least make the task more deliberative and effective, particularly in clinical situations involving multiple uncertainties with dire consequences. Paradoxically, it is in these situations that uncertainty is often most ineffectively addressed because of the extreme cognitive and emotional demands it places on clinicians and patients. It is easier for both clinicians and patients to simply "go with the flow" of medical intervention: to succumb to clinical inertia and medicine's "therapeutic imperative"[32] in lieu of directly confronting the specific uncertainties that are affecting them. A framework-guided approach to uncertainty management can help mitigate this problem by prompting clinicians and patients to pause and systematically take stock of their uncertainties and to address them in a more targeted, rational manner.

Consider the case of a seriously ill 70-year-old man with COVID-19 pneumonia, currently hospitalized in the intensive care unit (ICU) of a busy urban hospital. The patient has been on mechanical ventilation for 3 days and is now developing worsening hypoxemia and signs of multisystem organ failure. The patient's critical care physician and his family are trying to decide whether to withdraw ventilatory support and institute comfort measures only at this point or to initiate further life-sustaining therapies, including extracorporeal membrane oxygenation (ECMO) and hemodialysis. This is one of the most difficult, gut-wrenching types of situations in all of medicine, and uncertainty lies at the heart of it. The conscious awareness of ignorance causes both the physician and the family significant doubt, emotional distress, and decisional conflict.

The uncertainty that lies at the heart of this situation, however, is not a monolithic psychological state focused simply on the choice between two alternative courses of medical action. Packed within this uncertainty are numerous interconnected uncertainties that pertain to a variety of more specific issues—scientific, practical, and personal—that each exert their own effects. Scientific uncertainties include the patient's likelihood of survival with or without further life-sustaining therapies and the chances that his expected quality of life will be diminished if he survives the current hospitalization. Practical uncertainties include the ability of the patient's family members to spend meaningful time with their loved one given the hospital's isolation precautions. Personal uncertainties include the effects of the patient's illness and potential death on the psychological, social, and economic well-being of the patient's family. They also include moral uncertainties about the permissibility of withdrawing life-sustaining interventions and the appropriateness of devoting scarce ICU resources to this patient as opposed to others. Personal uncertainties also include existential uncertainties about the patient's preparedness for death and the alignment of his treatment plan with the kind of life or death that he would find meaningful and authentic. A final moral and existential uncertainty, which can have profound effects on the physician, the patient's family members, and loved ones alike, pertains to whether they have each done all they could to help the patient, professionally or personally. A framework-guided approach to uncertainty management can allow the physician and family to systematically account for these and other uncertainties and to establish their locus—that is, to determine in whose minds they reside. It can thus help ensure that important uncertainties are shared and addressed.

A framework-guided approach can also help clinicians and patients diagnose the sources of these uncertainties. The indeterminacy of future outcomes is a primary source of both scientific uncertainties about the patient's likelihood of survival and practical uncertainties about the well-being of the patient's family. In theory, this indeterminacy can be expressed in the form of objective, evidence-based probabilities. However, the current lack of scientific evidence on the outcomes of patients with COVID-19 makes these probabilities unknown—that is, ambiguous. Another important source of both the scientific and practical uncertainties of this patient's case, therefore, is not only the indeterminacy of various outcomes but also their indeterminability. This is also an important source of the physician's and family's personal uncertainties about the permissibility of withdrawing life-sustaining interventions, the appropriateness of ICU care, the patient's preparedness for death, the alignment between his care plan and his authentic values, and the adequacy of their own efforts to care for the patient. Objective, evidence-based probabilities for these personal uncertainties simply do not exist. Furthermore, the moral and existential nature of these uncertainties precludes the assignment of such probabilities to begin with: There is no single right answer or gold standard by which their accuracy could ever be assessed. The ultimate root cause of the moral and existential uncertainties in this case, therefore, is intractability. These uncertainties pertain to the most insoluble of all human mysteries: the meaning of good and evil, life and death, being and nonbeing. They are fundamentally resistant to complete comprehension and control.

A framework-guided approach to uncertainty management can next aid the physician and family in assessing the prognosis, or degree of reducibility, of their uncertainties. In the current case, scientific uncertainties about the patient's likelihood of survival and practical uncertainties about the impact of the patient's illness on the family's well-being are partially reducible by additional information. Personal uncertainties, in contrast, have a more guarded prognosis. Empirical evidence (e.g., prior documentation of the patient's preferences and values in an advanced directive or living will) might partially reduce uncertainties about the patient's preparedness for death and the acceptability of continued life-sustaining treatment. However, substantial uncertainty will always remain about how well individuals can know their own "true" values regarding such a ponderous, incomprehensible state as their own nonbeing—and how well any precertified piece of paper can adequately capture these values. These and other moral and existential uncertainties cannot be reduced by empirical evidence alone.

A framework-guided approach can next help clinicians and patients to determine appropriate, targeted treatments for the many uncertainties they are experiencing. The framework suggests a broad array of potential treatment options, both curative and palliative, and ignorance-, uncertainty-, response-, and person-focused (Chapter 4). Some options, such as ordering uncertainty (e.g., by classifying and categorizing or creating and following rules), are useful regardless of the individual or circumstance. Indeed, that is the fundamental premise of this book. Other options, such as adjusting uncertainty (e.g., by decreasing deliberation or ignoring ignorance), are essential for complex cases involving multiple uncertainties; human cognitive limitations prevent individuals from attending to all of them at once.

Beyond these basic treatment options, however, the appropriate strategies for managing any given uncertainty depend on its prognosis as well as the goals of management. For uncertainties that are reducible, cure is generally the primary goal, and ignorance-focused strategies are appropriate. In the current case, reducible scientific uncertainties about the patient's short-term outcomes might be treated by curative strategies, including information seeking (e.g., searching the medical literature for emerging evidence, performing additional laboratory testing or imaging studies that may have prognostic significance, or conducting a time-limited therapeutic trial of ECMO to assess the patient's immediate response). For uncertainties that are irreducible, the primary goal can only be palliation, and a variety of different palliative strategies—uncertainty-, response-, and person-focused—are possible and appropriate. In the current case, irreducible personal uncertainties about the morality of life-sustaining treatment and the patient's preparedness for death might be effectively treated by response-focused strategies such as adaptation (e.g., adjusting the goals of care to focus on ensuring the patient's physical, emotional, and spiritual well-being as opposed to his survival, or adjusting one's epistemic goals to relinquish the pursuit of absolute moral and existential certainty). Person-focused palliative strategies that might also be effective include self-affirmation (e.g., acknowledging core personal values of the patient and his family) and relating with others (e.g., fostering epistemic companionship and sharing decision-making responsibility between the healthcare team and members of the patient's family).

In many clinical situations, however, the goals and strategies for managing uncertainty are not so clear-cut. The uncertainty itself may be neither clearly reducible nor irreducible, or else the primary management goal may be neither cure nor palliation but some combination of the two, or something else altogether. In the current case prognostic uncertainty is incompletely reducible, and the primary goal of managing it is ambiguous. Although prognostic uncertainty is aversive for some patients and family members, it is psychologically necessary and morally desirable for many others confronting serious life-limiting illness, because it leaves open the possibility of a good outcome and thus serves the essential adaptive function of enabling hope.[33–36] In the current case, therefore, the primary goal may not be to "cure" or reduce prognostic uncertainty, but to maintain or even increase it through various strategies (e.g., increasing deliberation, highlighting ignorance due to the indeterminacy of future outcomes or ambiguity in available evidence).

A framework-guided approach to uncertainty management helps clarify how prognostic uncertainty itself can be palliative in nature and function, and that the optimal regulatory response may sometimes be to leave it alone. Doing so, however, requires the higher-order, metacognitive presence of mind to rise above and integrate both cure and palliation—to treat prognostic uncertainty not as an exclusively harmful phenomenon to be rejected and avoided, but as a simultaneously beneficial phenomenon to be accepted and embraced. In other words, the proper management of prognostic uncertainty ultimately requires uncertainty tolerance: the capacity to maintain one eye closed and one eye open—simultaneously pursuing management strategies aimed at both reducing uncertainty and its potential harms, and maintaining uncertainty and allowing the patient, his family, and his physician to derive benefit from it. A framework-guided approach alone does not confer this capacity; however, by prompting clinicians, patients, and family members to consider alternative goals and strategies for managing uncertainty, it creates the necessary conditions for uncertainty tolerance.

THE MANAGEMENT OF UNCERTAINTY: LIMITS AND POSSIBILITIES

The foregoing case study cannot possibly capture the full range of either the uncertainties that arise in medicine or the rich diversity of people's responses to them. However, I believe it illustrates both the value and the limitations of an integrative, framework-guided approach to uncertainty management. On the one hand, I have argued, such an approach can make this task more intentional, systematic, and goal directed. It can help clinicians and patients account for uncertainties, psychological responses, and regulatory strategies they might otherwise not have considered and make the management of these uncertainties more targeted and rational. It can enable individuals to identify the specific uncertainties that exist in a given medical situation and select and fashion management strategies that specifically address these uncertainties and their root causes—rather than taking a generic, one-size-fits-all approach.

On the other hand, a framework-guided approach offers no single right answers to the question of which specific management strategies—either curative or palliative, or ignorance-, uncertainty-, response-, or person-focused—are most appropriate for any given uncertainty, person, or situation. In the end, individual clinicians and patients must determine for themselves which management strategies are available and most appropriate based on their own unique experiences, values, and needs—details that were conspicuously absent in the foregoing case study. Furthermore, the inventory of strategies in the current framework is not exhaustive, and empirical evidence on their effectiveness in different situations is lacking. In these respects, the management of uncertainty parallels the management of other difficult medical problems: clinicians and patients must do the hard work of sorting through the particulars that make each case unique and manage uncertainty without really knowing whether their efforts will be successful. This is the art of medicine.

In other words, a framework-guided approach to uncertainty management requires—as well as aims for—UT. The managers of uncertainty must rise above the limits of their knowledge, come up with creative ways of adapting to these limits, and eventually move ahead. Humility, flexibility, and courage are the requisite capacities that enable each of these forms of transcendence. They help us see our uncertainty not only as a limitation but also as an opportunity, a space for all of us—clinicians, patients, and human beings—to create new possibilities and meanings. Humility, flexibility, and courage do not make uncertainty any less emotionally aversive or challenging to manage; however, they do free us from various self- and culturally imposed barriers to tolerating it. Humility frees us from the oppressive belief in single right answers and our ability to find them; it thus fosters ongoing openness toward new knowledge, respect for the views of others, and a willingness to revise our own views. Flexibility frees us from the stifling force of our own preconceptions and experiences; it thus enables us to consider alternative ways of dealing with our uncertainties and adapting to new challenges. Courage frees us from the fear of failure and imperfection; it thus permits us to relinquish our ultimately futile quest for absolute knowledge, to take a leap of faith when needed, and to accept the consequences. When approached with humility, flexibility, and courage, uncertainty becomes not only constraining but liberating.

The critical question is how to cultivate these vital capacities in clinical practice. One way, I believe, is to affirm the basic fallibility of all human knowledge, medical and otherwise. In my own personal experience on both sides of medical care—as a primary and palliative care physician, patient, and family member of seriously ill loved ones who have died—I have found that explicitly acknowledging my own ignorance and inability to know the "truth" makes the case for humility, flexibility, and courage obvious to all parties and sets a tone of UT. I have personally witnessed and felt, on both ends of the provider-patient relationship, how the tremendous emotional despair and angst caused by the uncertainty of serious illness can dissipate in response to the single admission that no one right answer exists, and that the task at hand is to work together to find the best answer we can based on the unavoidably imperfect knowledge we have. This admission is neither an abdication of personal responsibility to continue grappling with uncertainty nor an endorsement of an "anything goes" approach to it. On the contrary, it is an invitation to embrace our uncertainty and manage it with genuine humility, flexibility, and courage. It does not resolve dilemmas or lessen the pain of not knowing what to do or how things will end. But it does diminish the added, avoidable suffering caused by the tyranny of unrealistic epistemic expectations. Acknowledging the fallibility of our knowledge out loud is the first step in tolerating it.

Yet to truly promote UT in medicine, the requisite capacities of humility, flexibility, and courage need to be not only cultivated in individual interactions between clinicians and patients but also somehow built into the structures, processes, and culture of healthcare. In other words, UT needs to be systematized. In the next chapter I conclude this book by identifying various potential strategies for accomplishing this aim.

Chapter 6

A Way Forward

Systematizing Uncertainty Tolerance

A better appreciation and, in turn, a better management of uncertainty will not emerge out of more refined technical medical knowledge, but rather out of the physician's and patient's psyches where, after all, certainty and uncertainty are perceived, judged, evaluated, and prepared for expression. The attempt to moderate the defenses against the disregard of uncertainty is worth the effort for a number of reasons: (1) it would lighten physicians' burdens by absolving them from the responsibility for implicitly having promised more than they or medicine can deliver; (2) it would give patients a greater voice in decision-making; (3) it would greatly reduce the exploitation of unwarranted certainty for purposes of control rather than care; and (4) it would significantly reduce the feelings of psychological abandonment that patients experience whenever they sense that doctors are withdrawing behind a curtain of silence or evasion.

—Jay Katz[1]

In this book I have sketched the rough outlines of a framework for uncertainty tolerance: a conceptual guide that can enable clinicians and patients to achieve an optimal, adaptive balance of responses to the various uncertainties they experience in medicine. The framework consists of basic explanatory models of the nature, etiology, anatomy, and natural history of the uncertainties that arise in medicine and an

Uncertainty in Medicine. Paul K.J. Han, Oxford University Press. © Oxford University Press 2021.
DOI: 10.1093/oso/9780190270582.003.0006

integrative normative model for how these uncertainties might be managed. I have tried to show how a framework-guided approach to this effort can help individual clinicians and patients manage uncertainty in a more systematic, goal-directed manner and ultimately improve their capacity to tolerate uncertainty.

In this final chapter, I shift the focus of analysis from individual clinicians and patients to the healthcare system as a whole, to explore how uncertainty tolerance might be systematized—that is, built in to the structures, processes, and culture of medicine. Examining the three key capacities that need to be cultivated to promote uncertainty tolerance—humility, flexibility, and courage—I identify a few potential system-level strategies, encompassing medical practice, education, and research, that can be enacted to help achieve this goal (Figure 6.1). Strategies to foster humility include focused efforts aimed at increasing the communication of scientific uncertainty and cultivating epistemic maturity among clinicians and patients. Strategies to foster flexibility include efforts aimed at cultivating mindfulness and

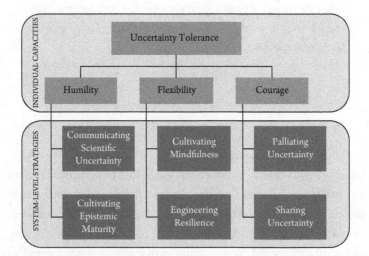

Figure 6.1 Systematizing uncertainty tolerance in medicine.

engineering resilience in the processes of healthcare. Finally, strategies to foster courage include focused efforts aimed at palliating the negative psychological effects of uncertainty and promoting sharing and collaborating in the management of uncertainty. I discuss the rationale for each of these strategies and show how they can help make uncertainty tolerance not an abstract ideal, but a normal way of thinking and being for clinicians and patients. I argue that these strategies can ultimately enable uncertainty tolerance to become part of both the worldview of individual clinicians and patients and the overarching culture of medicine. They can help expand the paradigm of medicine to focus not only on the pursuit of medical knowledge, but also on the equally important task of helping people live with uncertainty.

FOSTERING HUMILITY

The goal of system-level efforts to foster humility is to increase clinicians' and patients' awareness of inherent limits to medical knowledge and the need to accept these limits. Two potential strategies for achieving this goal include clinical and educational interventions aimed at (1) communicating scientific uncertainty and (2) cultivating epistemic maturity among clinicians and patients. These interventions ultimately aim to establish appropriate cognitive expectations about the attainability of medical knowledge.

Communicating scientific uncertainty. Effective communication of scientific uncertainty to and between clinicians, patients, and the general public is a primary strategy for fostering humility. Such communication prompts both parties to be aware of existing gaps in scientific knowledge, appropriately cautious in their judgments and decisions, and receptive to new evidence and information. Communicating scientific uncertainty is an essential element of shared decision-making, which not only allows patients to determine for themselves whether the existing level of scientific evidence warrants action, but also enables clinicians and patients to work collaboratively with one another as co-equal partners in deciding between "preference-sensitive" medical options.[2-6] Communicating scientific uncertainty places both clinicians and patients in a common space of humility that makes shared decision-making possible. In the public health domain, communicating scientific uncertainty can promote a healthy skepticism that may help health professionals and the lay public avoid both overconfidence and underconfidence in existing scientific evidence and recommendations.

The COVID-19 crisis has demonstrated how important this function is, yet how little is known about how to effectively communicate scientific uncertainty. Despite consensus on the importance of this effort, no empirically validated, standardized approaches to the task exist.[7-11] Not surprisingly, the most common approach of public health officials and government policymakers has been to simply describe both the COVID-19 threat and the recommended measures for reducing it without explicitly communicating scientific uncertainty about either issue. Although possibly motivated by beneficent intentions to minimize public fear or alarm, this disregard of uncertainty communication has had several unintended harms. It has promoted unwarranted certainty and unrealistic epistemic expectations that have not only prevented informed decision-making, but also created confusion and undermined public trust—particularly as new or conflicting scientific evidence or recommendations have emerged. Mask use, drug therapies (e.g., hydroxychloroquine, remdesivir, monoclonal antibody therapy), and vaccines have all been subject to conflicting and changing evidence and expert recommendations, which have subsequently generated significant public discord, distrust, and maladaptive behavior. A critical question is whether more explicit, consistent communication of scientific uncertainty by experts could have inoculated the public against such maladaptive reactions—averting inordinate confidence and uncritical acceptance of these interventions, as well as inordinate doubt and uncritical rejection when scientific evidence or opinion changes. By promoting epistemic humility, communicating scientific uncertainty may help both health professionals and laypersons respond to changing or conflicting information with greater equanimity.

Yet much remains unknown about how to effectively communicate scientific uncertainty to clinicians, patients, and the general public. Scientific research to address this knowledge gap is thus one important system-level strategy for promoting uncertainty tolerance. Most of what we know about communicating uncertainty has been derived from research conducted outside of medicine and focused on the communication of numeric estimates of risk, or probability—the primary representation of aleatory or first-order uncertainty arising from indeterminacy (Chapter 3). This work has shown that various ways of communicating risk information, including the use of visual representations, can improve comprehension.[12-17] In contrast, relatively little research has examined the communication of ambiguity—that is, the primary representation of epistemic or second-order uncertainty arising from indeterminability or intractability.[3,18,19] Methods of communicating ambiguity in probability estimates include the use of confidence intervals, risk ranges, best-case/worst-case options, or qualitative "hedging" language (e.g., "approximately," "about").[20] Although the general public is accustomed to some methods of communicating ambiguity (e.g., "margin of error" in opinion polls), there is wide variability in the use of similar expressions of imprecision in medical practice.[18,21] Methods of communicating ambiguity in other important types of scientific information, including the recommendations of scientific experts, include formalized language for rating the quality of scientific evidence. Examples include evidence rating schemes put forth by the US Preventive Services Task Force and the Grading of Recommendations Assessment, Development and Evaluation (GRADE) working group initiative.[22–24]

These and other approaches to communicating scientific uncertainty are not yet standardized, however, and many empirical questions remain regarding their effectiveness. A particularly important question pertains to the optimal level of precision in estimates of uncertainty. On the one hand, efforts to quantify probability and also ambiguity—that is, to assign precise, numeric estimates to our level of confidence in the occurrence of some medical unknown outcome—are increasing with the accumulation of empirical data and advances in predictive modeling methods. Greater quantitative precision in estimates of probability and ambiguity helps clarify the extent and nature of scientific uncertainty. However, its value for individual medical decisions is limited by the logical incoherence of using objective frequencies to describe the occurrence of single events.[25,26] At some point, furthermore, precision becomes psychologically irrelevant. Human reasoning is ultimately a "fuzzy" process based on imprecise, qualitative "gist representations"—as psychologist Valerie Reyna has called them—that capture the deeper, "bottom-line" meaning and significance of information.[27–29] Precise, quantitative "verbatim" representations, such as numeric estimates of probability or ambiguity, simply capture the surface form of phenomena, and often have secondary, instrumental importance in judgment and decision-making. An important question for future research is to determine how much informational precision is actually necessary for clinicians and patients to understand the gist meaning of the scientific uncertainties surrounding any given medical problem.[30] The broader need is to advance the science of uncertainty communication more generally and to determine which strategies are most appropriate for different individuals and situations.

System-level educational interventions to train health professionals to effectively communicate scientific uncertainty are a corollary need. Historically, this has not been a focus of either undergraduate or graduate medical education, and physicians thus lack competence in this task. The trend is shifting as educational programs in risk communication and shared decision-making are being developed and implemented by a growing number of medical schools and residency programs.[31-33] Much more work is needed, however, to disseminate these programs more broadly not only to physicians at various levels of training but also to nurses and other allied health professionals in various educational settings. Training in uncertainty communication for public health professionals has been part of broader training programs on risk communication, such as those developed by the US Centers for Disease Control and Prevention.[34] More work is needed to develop and disseminate training focused specifically on communicating the scientific uncertainties about public health risks and to harmonize strategies with those used in clinical as well as non-clinical settings.

Cultivating epistemic maturity. Effective communication of scientific uncertainty fosters humility and promotes uncertainty tolerance by cultivating what educational psychologists have called "epistemic maturity"—a developmental state characterized by epistemological beliefs, or "personal epistemologies," that acknowledge fundamental limits to human knowledge.[35-39] Epistemic maturity is thought to evolve over time with learning and experience— progressing from a naïve "dualistic" view of knowledge as right versus wrong, absolute, definitive, and stable, to a "relativistic" view of knowledge as pluralistic, context dependent, contingent, tentative, and mutable.[36,38,40-42] Epistemic maturity represents an advanced type of thinking that considers the limits and criteria of knowledge and is tentative and flexible in evaluating truth claims.[43,44]

An intriguing question is whether a lack of epistemic maturity may be responsible for aversive psychological responses to uncertainty— and conversely, whether the development of epistemic maturity may mitigate these responses. Decision scientist Robert Winkler has argued incisively that the well-described phenomenon of ambiguity aversion results from a mistaken epistemic belief in the existence of a single "true" objective probability for a future event and a discomfort with not knowing this probability.[45] In other words, ambiguity aversion may arise not only from a fear of what is not known, but also from unrealistic epistemic expectations about what can be known. Supporting this view, empirical studies have shown that correcting these naïve epistemic expectations—that is, reinforcing the unknowable nature of the probability of a given event—reduces ambiguity aversion.[46] It is possible, therefore, that fostering epistemic maturity (i.e., normalizing the inherent limits to knowledge) may help people tolerate uncertainty. Supporting this possibility, my colleagues and I have found that the addition of "uncertainty-normalizing" language to public health messages conveying scientific uncertainty about the COVID-19 pandemic reduces ambiguity-averse responses to these messages.[47]

The critical question is whether epistemic maturity can be intentionally cultivated in medicine. We lack a definitive empirical answer to this question; however, we do know that epistemic maturity among physicians is mutable. In her seminal ethnographic studies of medical school training, sociologist Renée Fox described how students learn to manage uncertainty by engaging in ignorance-focused strategies aimed at acquiring knowledge, as well as various response-focused strategies (e.g., humor, impiety, self-mockery, and "detached concern").[48-50] Yet the ultimate stage in the evolution of students' ability to manage medical uncertainty was the development of a kind of epistemic equanimity that Fox described vividly:

> Students gradually evolved what they referred to as a more "affirmative attitude" toward medical uncertainty. They became more able to accept uncertainty as inherent in medicine, to sort out their own

limitations from those of the field, meet uncertainty with candor, and to take a "positive, philosophy-of-doubting" approach. In clinical situations, they were more prone to feel and display sufficient "certitude" to make decisions and reassure patients.[48]

It thus seems possible to cultivate epistemic maturity, although the most effective strategies remain to be determined. Greater attention to this effort, however, is justified by the many potential negative effects of epistemic immaturity in medicine. An inability to acknowledge limits to medical knowledge can set clinicians and patients off on a relentless and futile pursuit of absolute certainty through overtesting and overtreatment. It can ultimately lead to professional burnout and both professional and patient dissatisfaction when perfect knowledge eventually proves unattainable.

Clinicians are a primary target for system-level efforts to cultivate epistemic maturity, and various educational efforts may promote this goal. Promising examples include training programs in evidence-based medicine and clinical reasoning in undergraduate medical education. More recently, innovative educational programs that support the development of epistemically mature beliefs and approaches to problem-solving have begun to make their way into medical school curricula. For example, training in visual thinking strategies[51-53] and improvisation[54,55] may help physician-trainees to develop skills in recognizing the subjectivity of their own perceptions and dealing with uncertainty, ambiguity, and surprise. Education in narrative medicine and medical humanities also supports the development of mature epistemic beliefs and thinking skills by challenging learners to understand differing viewpoints and perspectives and to question their own.[56,57] Physician and writer Danielle Ofri has argued that medical humanities education allows learners "to develop the underused mental muscles of reflection and contemplation" and can thereby help clinicians to "confront and relish ambiguity."[56] At the University of Arizona College of Medicine, surgeon and medical educator Marlys Witte has developed a "Curriculum on Medical Ignorance" that addresses medical uncertainty more specifically and explicitly. The goal of this program is to help undergraduate medical students "recognize and deal productively with ignorance, uncertainty, and the unknown," by building their skills in "raising, listening to, analyzing, prioritizing, and answering questions from different points of view."[58,59] The common feature of all of these promising educational programs is a focus on cultivating mature epistemic beliefs and problem-solving skills. More work is needed to further develop and refine these programs and to evaluate their effectiveness.

Patients and the general public are equally important targets for system-level efforts to cultivate epistemic maturity. Promising examples consist of public information campaigns designed to cultivate epistemic maturity, such as the Choosing Wisely® initiative of the ABIM Foundation[60] and emerging efforts to educate the public about overdiagnosis and overtreatment.[61,62] These efforts aim to promote healthy skepticism about medical interventions and to teach laypersons to critically assess their value before accepting them. More concerted efforts like these are needed to shift the "epistemic culture" of medicine—to borrow the term coined by sociologist Karin Knorr Cetina[63]—toward greater humility and tolerance of uncertainty.

FOSTERING FLEXIBILITY

The goal of system-level efforts to foster flexibility is to increase clinicians' and patients' capacity to adjust and rebalance their diverse, often conflicting, responses to uncertainty to adapt to changing circumstances. Two potential strategies for achieving this goal are (1) promoting mindfulness and (2) engineering resilience, both of which paradoxically aim to make flexibility a consistent, habitual aspect of medical care.

Cultivating mindfulness. One important strategy for fostering flexibility is rooted in the notion of "reflective practice," a meta-cognitive process "whereby an individual thinks analytically about anything relating to their professional practice with the intention of gaining insight and using the lessons learned to maintain good practice or make improvements where possible."[64] Increasingly promoted as a means of improving healthcare quality and safety, reflective practice also plays a broader role in the management of uncertainty. Philosopher Donald Schön viewed the central function of reflective practice, which he termed "reflection-in-action," as enabling people to "make new sense of the situations of uncertainty or uniqueness"[65] by prompting them to question their tacit understandings, to become aware of other ways of framing reality, and to adapt their approaches the particular uncertainties at hand.[65]

Physician, researcher, and educator Ron Epstein expanded the meaning and scope of this process in his concept of mindfulness, which he defined as both a "discipline and attitude of mind" that enables one "to become more aware of one's own mental processes, listen more attentively, become flexible, and recognize bias and judgments, and thereby act with principles and compassion."[66] In this sense mindfulness represents a positive attitude toward uncertainty, an orientation toward maintaining and benefiting from it. Borrowing a concept put forth by Zen Buddhist practitioner Shunryu Suzuki Roshi, Epstein likened mindfulness to the attainment of "beginner's mind"—a "cultivated naïveté" in which one attempts to suspend judgment and to question and set aside one's prior knowledge and preconceptions in order to see a situation in new ways and from different perspectives.[67,68] Mindfulness entails a sense of "unfinished-ness" in one's orientation to the world, a posture of humility and curiosity regarding one's incomplete understanding of the suffering of another.[66] More than a mere acknowledgment of ignorance, however, mindfulness represents an affirming response to it—a capacity to see new possibilities in incomplete understanding—which ultimately enables clinicians to tolerate uncertainty. Mindfulness could be characterized as a means of cultivating all three of the key capacities that comprise uncertainty tolerance—humility, flexibility, and courage. However, I believe its role in cultivating flexibility is especially important; mindfulness enables individuals to self-monitor and regulate their own responses to uncertainty. Epstein argued that for practicing clinicians, mindfulness promotes the cognitive flexibility to let go of ideas when they are no longer useful, and to adapt to the inherent ambiguities and contradictions posed by patients and patient care.[68]

The larger, unanswered question is how best to cultivate mindfulness in healthcare. Epstein and colleagues have developed health professional training workshops on mindfulness, and empirical evidence supports their effectiveness in promoting physician well-being and attitudes toward patient-centered care.[67,69,70] Epstein has also outlined a set of basic mindfulness practices that clinicians can employ in their daily practices. Examples include pausing momentarily before a patient encounter in order to collect one's thoughts, become present in the moment, and let go of expectations. One can then ask oneself reflective, "opening-up" questions that help identify one's own cognitive blind spots: "Is there another way to view this situation? What am I assuming that might not be true? How are prior experiences and expectations affecting how I view the situation? What would a trusted peer say?"[68] Formal reflective practice training programs have also begun to be developed and implemented in undergraduate and graduate medical education; some of these have focused specifically on medical uncertainty (e.g., using reflective writing exercises and critical thinking activities).[71–73] System-level reflective practice interventions have also been implemented in clinical settings as a means of improving healthcare safety and quality. Examples include formal case review exercises, daily huddles, and other structured team interactions aimed at promoting self-reflection and flexibility in solving problems. Although implemented for different specific purposes, all of these initiatives have the same fundamental outcome of promoting mindfulness among clinicians and flexibility in approaching medical problems. Most importantly, they offer the opportunity to achieve the somewhat paradoxical goal of systematizing mindfulness—making it a more automatic and routine part of medical care.

Engineering resilience. Another promising strategy for fostering flexibility has been put forth by the "resilient healthcare" (RHC) movement,[74,75] an effort to apply systems engineering principles to improve resilience—which health systems scientists Erik Hollnagel, Jeffrey Braithwaite, and Robert Wears have defined as the healthcare system's ability to "adjust its functioning prior to, during, or following changes and disturbances, so that it can sustain required performance under both expected and unexpected conditions."[74] The defining attribute of resilience is flexibility—that is, the "capacity to switch from one strategy to another" and "to select the most appropriate strategy"[76] that allows the system to remain intact and functional despite the presence of threats.[75] RHC views healthcare as a complex adaptive system that is fundamentally indeterminate, intractable, and unpredictable due to multiplicity in its elements and interactions, nonlinear effects and feedback loops, emergent properties, self-organization, learning, and evolution.[77,78] The epistemological implication of this view is that uncertainty in healthcare must be accepted and approached with flexibility. As physician and health services researcher Trisha Greenhalgh put it: "There are no universal solutions to the challenges of complex health systems, nor is there a set of universal methods that will bring us closer to the truth."[79] Therefore, efforts to understand and improve healthcare quality must focus not on eliminating variation, surprise, and uncertainty in everyday work, but on adapting to them.[74,77]

Toward this end, RHC interventions aim to promote four key capacities in the healthcare system: (1) Respond to everyday work and unexpected events as they arise; (2) monitor and understand current work processes; (3) learn from past experience; and (4) anticipate challenges in order to prevent or mitigate their effects.[77,80] Unlike "Safety-I" approaches to improving healthcare quality and safety, which are reactively focused on identifying and eliminating adverse events and their causes,[77] RHC focuses on "Safety-II" approaches, which are proactively focused on improving a system's overall capacity to maximize acceptable outcomes.[80] Such approaches include real-time data and information feedback processes; statistical modeling to predict and simulate alternative outcomes; contingency plans; and care process redesign to facilitate interaction, information sharing, and trust building.[81]

Kathleen Sutcliffe and Karl Weick have characterized RHC as a process of "mindful organizing" involving attention to context and capacities to act, which allows systems "to marshal the necessary resources and capabilities to act on that understanding in a flexible manner that is tailored to the unexpected contingency."[82]

Resilient healthcare interventions ultimately aim to redesign the structures and processes of healthcare to promote resilient attitudes, values, behaviors, and practices, which then become part of a new organizational culture—a "taken for granted, 'normal' way of being and doing."[83] As Hollnagel, Braithwaite, and Wears have argued, RHC does not consist of a single, specifiable set of outcomes, given that resilience itself represents a capacity rather than a particular state:

> It is practically impossible to specify precisely what resilient perfor-
> mance will look like, and therefore also directly to engineer it. The
> adjustments that people make—the trade-offs and "sacrifices"—are

the results of individual or collective decision making rather than an engineered feature. . . . Performance, successes and failures alike, requires the ability to adjust in the given situation in a measured, thoughtful way that characterizes smooth adaptation to the system's challenges.[84]

The concept of resilience in healthcare and the concept of uncertainty tolerance thus share important features. Just as it is impossible to specify what uncertainty tolerance looks like for any given individual, problem, and situation, so it is with resilient—that is, flexible—performance. RHC, like uncertainty tolerance, is not a state that can be prespecified or directly engineered, but rather a capacity to adjust and adapt to the unique demands of a given situation. Both RHC and uncertainty tolerance rest on the epistemological premise that medical ignorance is fundamentally irreducible, and that surprise and variation in healthcare outcomes are thus unavoidable. They are both ideal states that ultimately require the flexibility to see ignorance as a source of new opportunities and to act upon them. As systems scientists Reuben McDaniel and Dean Driebe have put it eloquently:

If the assumption is that surprise often arises as the result of the fundamental unknowability of the world, we open the door for creative, innovative approaches without the mark of blame and failure. We change our relationship with the unexpected and resilience becomes a quality that is essential for effective management. Surprise seen negatively (as error) often leads to a search for reliability whereas surprise seen positively (as opportunity) can led to a search for new approaches to situations.[85]

In the broadest sense, the ideal of RHC amounts to uncertainty tolerance at the health system level. RHC interventions represent efforts to systematize uncertainty tolerance by changing our "relationship with the unexpected," institutionalizing the flexibility needed to treat surprise positively, as an opportunity for new management approaches.

FOSTERING COURAGE

The goal of system-level efforts to foster courage is to increase clinicians' and patients' psychological and existential capacity to move forward with their lives in spite of their uncertainty and its negative effects. Two potential strategies for achieving this goal are (1) palliating uncertainty and (2) sharing uncertainty, which focus, respectively, on providing the emotional and relational support needed to tolerate uncertainty.

Palliating uncertainty. A primary system-level strategy for fostering courage is to palliate uncertainty—that is, to ameliorate the psychological suffering it causes for both patients and clinicians. Historically, this task has received little attention; consistent with medicine's approach to most other problems, the focus has been on curative rather than palliative care. In recent years, however, promising strategies for palliating uncertainty have begun to emerge and may provide the basis for further efforts to advance the science and practice of uncertainty palliation.

One set of strategies consists of uncertainty-focused psychotherapeutic interventions developed to treat anxiety disorders. A prime example is an intervention, known as cognitive behavior therapy targeting intolerance of uncertainty (CBT-IU), which utilizes cognitive behavioral therapy (CBT) targeted specifically at individuals' intolerance of uncertainty.[86–88] Developed by clinical psychologists Melisa Robichaud, Naomi Koerner, and Michel Dugas to treat generalized anxiety disorder and related conditions, CBT-IU uses psychoeducation and training to teach people to reduce the excessive, maladaptive worry prompted by uncertainty and their propensity toward catastrophic interpretations in response to uncertainty-inducing situations.[89-94] Its ultimate goal is to help patients achieve a "less negative, more balanced perspective on the threat of uncertainty in their daily lives" by teaching them to recognize their worry and its relationship to uncertainty, reevaluate the usefulness of worry, reappraise problems, and ultimately reevaluate their catastrophic interpretations about uncertainty and its consequences.[86] The intervention equips patients with the metacognitive self-awareness and skills to serve as their own therapists who can manage and tolerate their own uncertainty.[89,95] Studies have demonstrated CBT-IU to be effective although time and resource intensive, and so far its use has been restricted to individuals with pathological levels of anxiety and worry. Other promising CBT-based interventions include *metacognitive therapy*, which aims at promoting "detached mindfulness" (a capacity to "stand back from" and disengage from worry or maladaptive responses to uncertainty[96]) and *acceptance and commitment therapy*, which aims to increase psychological flexibility[97] and reduce avoidant coping behaviors by promoting "acceptance, mindfulness, flexible attention to the now, and cognitive defusion."[98]

Existential therapy is another promising CBT approach focused on helping people respond to important life threat by enhancing their ability to find meaning and affirm fundamental values.[99, 100] Rooted in insights from European existential philosophy, this approach has a long history. It focuses on helping individuals overcome fundamental anxieties about their own mortality and limited knowledge and control of their lives by accepting and transcending these conditions. Psychiatrist Viktor Frankl argued that underlying these fundamental anxieties is a "will to meaning"—a basic human drive to discover values or ideals that provide a sense of meaning in life—and that achieving this sense of meaning is what allows individuals to transcend their limitations and move ahead with their lives.[101] In a similar vein, existentialist theologian Paul Tillich argued that faith—in the sense of being "grasped" by some "ultimate concern" that makes life meaningful—is what allows individuals to transcend their limitations and to overcome the anxieties that arise from an awareness of these limitations.[102] It gives people the "courage to be" in spite of the threat of nonbeing. Rollo May, a pioneer in the field of existential psychology, further refined Tillich's conception and viewed psychotherapy as enabling people to create the meaning they need to face their anxieties and realize their potential in life.[103]

The critical question is whether elements of these or other psychotherapeutic approaches are feasible and effective in the broader context of medical practice, and accumulating evidence suggests that this may be the case. Existential therapy has been the basis of a "meaning-centered psychotherapy" program for advanced cancer patients, developed by psychiatrist William Breitbart and colleagues,[104] while nursing scholar Merle Mishel and colleagues have developed a CBT-based intervention to help breast cancer survivors cope with the uncertainty and fear of cancer recurrence.[105] "Dignity therapy," a brief meaning-focused bedside intervention developed by psychiatrist Harvey Chochinov to treat psychological distress among seriously ill patients at the end of life, has also been shown to improve coping.[106,107] These successful efforts suggest the potential value of CBT and other psychotherapeutic strategies in palliating the negative effects of uncertainty for individuals without pathological emotional disorders.

All of these interventions promote courage by palliating the aversive psychological effects of uncertainty that prevent people from moving forward and living with the unknown. The larger question is whether the "active ingredients" of these interventions—the key elements that ameliorate the negative effects of uncertainty—can be isolated, and whether more effective interventions focused specifically on palliating uncertainty can be developed and implemented in diverse clinical practice settings. Broader dissemination and implementation will likely require briefer interventions that can feasibly be undertaken at the bedside by various types of clinicians. Further research to develop, implement, and evaluate such interventions, and to advance both the science and practice of uncertainty palliation more generally, is an important system-level need.

Sharing uncertainty. Another promising system-level strategy for fostering courage is to institutionalize the sharing of uncertainty among clinicians and patients. This strategy is an extension of growing health system initiatives to advance interprofessional team care, "shared care," and "collaborative care."[108-110] These initiatives aim to improve healthcare quality by enhancing the sharing of knowledge and task responsibilities among health professionals from different disciplines (e.g., medicine, nursing, social work, pharmacy, physical and occupational therapy). The primary focus of these initiatives is to increase communication, care coordination, and teamwork as a means of decreasing team members' uncertainty about both the problem at hand and their roles in managing it. In her theory of "relational coordination," management scientist Jody Hoffer Gittell argued that effective, efficient team functioning depends on a "mutually reinforcing process of communicating and relating for the purpose of task integration," and that central to this process is a sharing of knowledge, goals, and mutual respect between team members. She argued that this interprofessional sharing reduces team members' uncertainty about how to manage a problem, and its importance thus increases as the uncertainty associated with a problem increases.[111,112]

These initiatives, however, improve team functioning and the quality of healthcare by sharing not only knowledge but also uncertainty, and by not only reducing uncertainty but also helping team members to comanage it. A shared consciousness of what team members do not know is as integral to high-quality, team-based care as a shared consciousness of what they do know; it helps them to then formulate a plan for reducing reducible uncertainties, and collectively managing irreducible ones. Sharing uncertainty fosters courage among team members by distributing the burden of uncertainty, which include not only its negative psychological effects but also the practical, moral, and legal responsibilities for managing it. The achievement of shared uncertainty deserves greater emphasis in system-level initiatives to institutionalize team, shared, and collaborative care.

Shared uncertainty is also integral to growing health system initiatives aimed at improving patient-centered care. It is a key element of shared decision-making—a process of "collaborative deliberation," as physician and researcher Glyn Elwyn has put it, in which clinicians and patients exchange information about medical options and work together to make decisions consistent with patients' values and preferences.[4-6] In this idealized process, the sharing of uncertainty about existing options enables patients to make better informed decisions that account for the quality of the available evidence.[113] To enable decision-making, however, efforts to promote shared decision-making cannot stop at simply sharing uncertainty in an informational sense. Uncertainty normally has a disabling effect on decision-making; this is the crux of the well-established psychological phenomenon of ambiguity aversion. To enable decision-making, efforts to promote shared decision-making must thus share uncertainty in a broader emotional, relational, moral, and existential sense. They must help the patient and clinician achieve what Ron Epstein and health communication researcher Richard Street have called "shared mind": an interactive state involving the sharing of "thoughts, feelings, perceptions, meanings, and intentions among 2 or more people."[114] This requires not only exchanging information, but also facilitating what Epstein and Street called "attunement"—a feeling of "being on the same wavelength or in stride with another person."[114] Shared mind also requires establishing interpersonal relationships of mutual trust and distributing moral responsibility for decision-making between both parties. At a more fundamental level, it requires providing "epistemic companionship" to one another, which creates a therapeutic sense of "generalized shared reality."[115] The very presence of another human being alleviates existential isolation and encourages individuals who are facing the unknown.[116]

I believe it is the sharing of uncertainty in this broader, deeper sense, which is not strictly informational but personal and relational, that provides clinicians and patients with the courage to overcome their natural tendency toward ambiguity aversion and to move forward and make difficult decisions in spite of it. If this is true, then system-level efforts to promote shared decision-making should devote greater attention to the noninformational processes involved in sharing uncertainty. At a practical level, this means not only developing and implementing decision support tools that convey information to patients, but also redesigning the structures and processes of healthcare to promote meaningful patient-clinician interactions and relationships and to provide patients with greater levels of psychological and social support. Potential approaches include new models of care, such as the Veterans Affairs Whole Health System initiative,[117] which aims to promote patient empowerment, self-care, and care integration by utilizing transdisciplinary teams and expanding access to health promotion and supportive care services. System changes like this are needed to expand the focus of shared decision-making interventions beyond information exchange alone.

A BRAVE NEW WORLDVIEW

So far as man stands for anything, and is productive or originative at all, his entire vital function may be said to have to deal with maybes. Not a victory is gained, not a deed of faithfulness or courage is done, except upon a maybe; not a service, not a sally of generosity, not a scientific exploration or experiment or textbook, that may not be a mistake. It is only by risking our persons from one hour to another that we live at all. And often enough our faith beforehand in an uncertified result is the only thing that makes the result come true. . . . as the essence of courage is to stake one's life on a possibility, so the essence of faith is to believe that the possibility exists.[118]

—William James

I have offered a few tentative ideas for how uncertainty tolerance might be systematized—that is, built into the routine structures, processes, and culture of medicine, so that it can become a normal way of acting and being for clinicians and patients. I have identified various system-level strategies aimed at fostering humility, flexibility, and courage, the higher-level vital capacities, or "be goals" needed to achieve an optimal, adaptive balance of responses to uncertainty. These strategies span medical care, education, and research, and I have argued that they provide a promising foundation for future efforts to systematize uncertainty tolerance.

This list of strategies, however, is by no means exhaustive. It does not include increasingly influential interventions aimed at increasing the precision of medical knowledge, such as the application of genome sequencing and editing technologies and of "big data," predictive analytics, and artificial intelligence to various medical problems. The strategies I have outlined also do not directly address several important barriers to uncertainty tolerance, encompassing not fear of malpractice liability but various broader cultural, social, and political factors that influence the construction of ignorance and our awareness of and responses to it. Examples include a growing antiscience movement, expanding dissemination of misinformation and disinformation through various media channels, increasing social and political polarization, and structural inequalities in access to healthcare. The negative influence of these factors on both our collective uncertainty and our responses to it have been on full display during the COVID-19 pandemic.

Nevertheless, I believe the limited set of strategies I have proposed provides a useful starting point for broader efforts to shift medicine toward a new, expanded paradigm—one that focuses not only on pursuing knowledge but on helping people live with uncertainty. In the final analysis, however, such a paradigm shift entails a prior, deeper philosophical commitment. The approach I have put forth both begins and ends in a more fundamental worldview consisting of particular ontological, epistemological, and moral preconceptions. In this worldview, reality is fundamentally indeterminate, human knowledge is inherently limited, and right action is contingent on the particulars of the individual and situation. These conceptions are built in to the framework I have presented; they suggest a particular way of thinking about uncertainty that itself allows one to accept and reconcile the paradoxes of uncertainty and our responses to it. Together, they form a worldview of uncertainty tolerance.

This worldview itself, furthermore, is not new. It was originally—and I believe most eloquently—articulated over a century ago by philosopher, psychologist, and physician William James. From an ontological standpoint, James viewed "indeterminism" as a given; he argued that events in the universe "have a certain amount of loose play on one another, so that the laying down of one of them does not necessarily determine what the others shall be," and that "things not yet revealed to our knowledge may really in themselves be ambiguous."[119] But James's uncertainty-tolerant response was to view indeterminism not strictly as a limitation or source of fear, but as a "gift" that makes life meaningful.[119] For James, indeterminism meant that reality is not "ready-made and complete from all eternity," but rather "still in the making"—unfinished and full of possibility.[120]

From an epistemological standpoint, James understood human knowledge as inherently limited and truth as fundamentally pluralistic. As he put it, "no single point of view can ever take in the whole scene."[120] But James's uncertainty-tolerant response to the absence of single right answers, and absolute truth was a philosophy of "pragmatism," which focused on judging the validity of any understanding of reality according to its practical consequences. For James, pragmatism was not a definitive philosophical system but an attitude or orientation: "The attitude of looking away from first things, principles, 'categories,' supposed necessities; and of looking toward last things, fruits, consequences, facts."[120] James's pragmatism was a plea for intellectual humility, practicality, and openness and "against dogma, artificiality, and the pretence of finality in truth." In James's view, pragmatism was a means of loosening and relativizing our beliefs and theories while viewing them as essential mental modes of adaptation to reality.[120]

> Theories thus become instruments, not answers to enigmas, in which we can rest. We don't lie back on them, we move forward, and, on occasion, make nature over again by their aid. Pragmatism unstiffens all our theories, limbers them up and sets each one at work.... It lies in the midst of our theories, like a corridor in a hotel. Innumerable chambers open out of it. In one you may find a man writing an atheistic volume; in the next some one on his knees praying for faith and strength; in a third a chemist investigating a body's properties. In a fourth a system of idealistic metaphysics is being excogitated; in a fifth the impossibility of metaphysics is being shown. But they all own the corridor, and all must pass through it if they want a practicable way of getting into or out of their respective rooms.[120]

From a moral standpoint, James acknowledged the difficulty of supplying particular answers to the question of right conduct in life; of pragmatism, he specified that "at the outset, at least, it stands for no particular results" (emphasis mine). However, his uncertainty-tolerant response was an openness to faith in some guiding ideal in life, which he saw as a necessary part of living.[121] A genuine pragmatist, argued James, "is willing to live on a scheme of uncertified possibilities which he trusts; willing to pay with his own person, if need be, for the realization of the ideals which he frames."[122] In other words, although pragmatism supplies the humility, practicality, and openness needed to consider alternative possibilities for action in the face of uncertainty, it is not sufficient; faith is also necessary.[121]

And often enough our faith beforehand in an uncertified result is the only thing that makes the result come true. Suppose, for instance, that you are climbing a mountain, and have worked yourself into a position from which the only escape is by a terrible leap. Have faith that you can successfully make it, and your feet are nerved to its accomplishment. But mistrust yourself, and think of all the sweet things you have heard the scientists say of maybes, and you will hesitate so long that at last, all unstrung and trembling, and launching yourself in a moment of despair, you roll in the abyss. In such a case (and it belongs to an enormous class), the part of wisdom as well as of courage is to believe what is in the line of your needs, for only by such belief is the need fulfilled. Refuse to believe, and you shall indeed be right, for you shall irretrievably perish. But believe, and again you shall be right, for you shall save yourself. You make one or the other of two possible universes true by your trust or mistrust—both universes having been only maybes, in this particular, before you contributed your act.[118]

An important leitmotif throughout James's work was thus an affirmation of faith as an existential need. Consistent with his pragmatism, James did not advocate for faith in any particular human ideal. The one exception, however, was faith in a better world and its attainability through human action. James called this particular faith "meliorism," by which he meant a brave "moral optimism"—a belief that desirable outcomes in life are neither inevitable nor impossible, but rather possible to attain.[120,122] James saw faith in this possibility—that "the future may be other and better than the past has been"—as providing not only the basis for courage, but also the very reason for living. As he put it, "A world with a chance in it of being altogether good, even if the chance never come to pass, is better than a world with no such chance at all. . . . This is the only chance we have any motive for supposing to exist."[119]

An indeterminate conception of reality that construes the universe as unfinished and full of possibility; a fallibilistic conception of knowledge as pluralistic and constructed, and truth as a function of its practical consequences; an individually focused and optimistic conception of right belief and action as requiring a self-fulfilling faith in the possibility of a better world: These are the philosophical commitments inherent to the concept of uncertainty tolerance. They comprise a coherent worldview that enables us to reconcile our simultaneous aversion and attraction to uncertainty and to balance our conflicting psychological responses to it. They turn uncertainty on its head, casting it in the same positive light—as enabling, empowering, and necessary—that we view knowledge.[120]

This brave, uncertainty-tolerant worldview that James articulated at the turn of the twentieth century contrasts with the worldview of modern medicine, which treats human knowledge as theoretically unlimited, reality as deterministic, and knowledge—the understanding of what is "right"—as our ultimate goal. This rational, uncertainty-averse worldview has certainly fueled great medical progress and found its ultimate expression in the aspirational ideal of "precision medicine." At the same time, however, I believe this worldview has also been maladaptive. It has fostered unrealistic epistemic expectations that set us up for failure, disappointment, and ever more aversive responses to uncertainty. It has prevented us from attending to these responses and their effects on our well-being.

Systematizing uncertainty tolerance in medicine, I believe, ultimately requires breaking this vicious cycle by adopting a new worldview. It requires recognizing the fundamental indeterminacy of all medical conditions, the insurmountable limits of all medical knowledge, and the inescapable need for faith in all medical decisions and actions. It requires seeing uncertainty as an integral aspect of all human knowledge—a metacognitive state that serves essential functions—as opposed to the mere absence of knowledge. It requires reframing medical uncertainty as a normal part of human life that must be adapted to, as opposed to a pathological state that must be cured.

A worldview alone cannot make individual clinicians and patients more tolerant of uncertainty; however, I believe it can help. By explicitly affirming the reasons why uncertainty is an irreducible and necessary part of medicine, an uncertainty-tolerant worldview can foster the development of a new collective mindset that can change our approach to the problem. It can empower clinicians and patients to more openly admit their uncertainty and to work together to manage it. It can also motivate researchers, administrators, and policymakers to prioritize medical uncertainty as a problem and to develop and implement more effective, evidence-based uncertainty management strategies. At a broader, cultural level, an uncertainty-tolerant worldview can help establish a different ethos for medical care, expanding its mission from simply abolishing or curing medical uncertainty to helping people live with it. Articulating such a worldview is thus a critical step toward systematizing uncertainty tolerance in medicine.

Importantly, a worldview of uncertainty tolerance does not disvalue the pursuit of medical knowledge or undermine the ideal of precision medicine. The pursuit of knowledge is and always will be the central focus of medicine. At a collective, macro level, we desperately need to know how to put a stop to the COVID-19 pandemic and countless other threats to human health and life. At an individual, micro level, each one of us needs to know—as precisely as we can—how to stay healthy, to avert disease and suffering, to forestall death, and to preserve the well-being of our families and loved ones. But in the end, we always return to the same problem: What do we do in the meantime, while we watchfully wait for the knowledge we need? How do we live with our uncertainty? This problem takes us out of the realm of knowledge and into the realm of other fundamental human capacities. These capacities include not only humility, flexibility, courage, but also faith—not only in the possibility of something better, but also in fundamental, "ultimate concerns"[101] that make life meaningful and help us transcend our human limitations. Fostering these capacities calls for nonmedical interventions that remain to be discovered; however, the point is that such efforts do not supplant the pursuit of medical knowledge but rather supplement it. Helping people live with uncertainty is a parallel endeavor of medical care.

In this sense, adopting a worldview of uncertainty tolerance increases—rather than decreases—precision in medicine by helping clinicians and patients respond to uncertainty in a more targeted, appropriate manner. It encourages them to pursue knowledge when medical ignorance is reducible, but to forgo this pursuit when ignorance is irreducible or even desirable from a psychological or existential standpoint. In such situations, an uncertainty-tolerant worldview can help clinicians and patients achieve the presence of mind to shift from curing to palliating medical uncertainty—to enact response- and person-focused management strategies that are more emotional and relational than cognitive in nature and aimed at minimizing the harms and maximizing the benefits of uncertainty. It allows them the freedom to tailor these strategies to their own unique needs and circumstances.

BEYOND UNCERTAINTY IN MEDICINE

This book has been an effort to make sense of the problem of medical uncertainty. In this effort I have synthesized theoretical insights and empirical evidence from various thinkers and disciplines and presented a series of conceptual frameworks aimed at helping us to approach uncertainty and its management in a systematic, integrative manner. I have ventured well beyond the domain of medical science and practice in this effort, and necessarily so. For as I have tried to show, the uncertainties that arise in medicine are not strictly medical, and the same holds true for their solutions. Every time we attempt to manage medical uncertainty, we are pushing back against the entire universe—challenging its fundamental indeterminacy, indeterminability, and intractability. We are defying human nature—attempting to alter our basic cognitive, emotional, and behavioral responses to the unknown. We are resisting reality—rejecting the way things are in favor of the way we want them to be. Eventually, however, we come to realize that in spite of our best efforts we are never completely successful; our knowledge and control of our health and destiny are limited. Medical uncertainty is thus ultimately not a medical but an existential problem that we must manage not by rejecting and resisting, but by accepting and transcending it: rising above our limited knowledge, crossing over our diverse psychological responses to our ignorance, and moving forward from the possible to the actual.

This multidimensional capacity to transcend uncertainty—to achieve a higher state of metauncertainty—is what the entire book has been about and what it aspires to promote. In the final analysis, the frameworks I have put forth are simply instruments of transcendence. Although they offer no single, definitive prescription for what we ought to do in any given medical situation, they provide a mental map and moral compass: a set of guiding principles that help us rise above our uncertainty so that we can begin to manage and tolerate it. At perhaps no other time in modern history has this task been more important. The COVID-19 pandemic has demonstrated beyond a shadow of a doubt how much human suffering and damage medical uncertainty can cause and how important it is to find a way to handle this uncertainty with equanimity: to keep one eye open and one eye closed, to avoid both excessive indifference and excessive panic.

When we transcend uncertainty, we put an end to uncertainty as we typically know it. We are able to treat uncertainty not as a discrete, pathological, maladaptive state of mind, but an integral, normal, adaptive state of being. We are able to approach it not as an obstacle to knowledge and object of tolerance, but a form of knowledge and inseparable aspect of tolerance itself. We are liberated from the tyranny of unrealistic expectations about the existence of single right answers and our ability to find them and freed to move forward in spite of our ignorance. When we transcend uncertainty, we see it as an inescapable, shared part of the human condition. We are able to openly acknowledge our uncertainty and commiserate about its effects, to empathize, to both give and receive help—that is, to actually care for one another. When we transcend uncertainty, we see it not as an obstacle closing us off from what we can know, but a door opening us up to what we can be. We are able to look beyond medicine itself, to the ultimate concerns that are the source of faith and meaning in our lives.

This is the profound paradox of uncertainty: It represents both our greatest liability and our greatest asset. It is both the bane of our existence and the precondition for a meaningful life. It brings us to our knees, but in doing so it brings out the best in us. The core problem of medicine and our lives more generally is to somehow accommodate this paradox: to maintain our uncertainty even as we strive to increase our knowledge and to derive benefit from it even as we experience—and strive to mitigate—its harms. For this problem I have offered no single definitive way forward, only some initial stepping stones for a journey into the unknown. But that means there are new possibilities still lying ahead of us, just waiting to be realized.

ACKNOWLEDGMENTS

This book would not have been possible without the encouragement and support of many people, to whom I am deeply grateful. Chad Zimmerman at Oxford University Press set things in motion 5 years ago, when he reached out about writing the book. He gave me the courage to start the project, and his kind, steadfast support helped keep it going. Sarah Humphreville took the reins after Chad moved on from OUP and provided valuable feedback on later drafts of the manuscript. I'm grateful for their confidence and patience through many missed deadlines. My writing ended up being interrupted not only by the usual professional and personal responsibilities of everyday life, but by significant, unanticipated events, including the death of my father and, most recently, a global pandemic that has turned all of our lives upside down. As painful as these events were and still are, they broadened my perspective on medical uncertainty and helped me write a different—it is hoped better—book. They gave me a visceral understanding of how uncertainty is both an affliction and a need, a source of both despair and hope, and that tolerating uncertainty means reconciling these dualities.

But many other persons and experiences have had an equally great influence on me over the years and have made this book a lifetime project. First and foremost were my parents, Dorothy Sang Ye Han and James Sun Nam Han, to whose memory I dedicate this book. Deeply religious first-generation Korean immigrants who began a new life in a terra incognita—my father was a Protestant minister who served several small-town parishes in the Midwest—my parents lived lives of humility, faith, and devotion to ideals beyond themselves. They taught me, by example, what it means to tolerate uncertainty and kindled my interest in fundamental questions of meaning in life and the limits of knowledge. These questions later motivated me to major in religious studies in college, where I came across the writings of William James, Paul Tillich, Keiji Nishitani, John Dewey, Peter Berger, Viktor Frankl, and many other thinkers who have had a lasting influence on my own worldview. I am grateful for the guidance of several teachers during this part of my journey, including A. Thomas Kirsch, Bernard Faure, and William Provine. When I later became a practicing general internist, my interest in questions of meaning and the limits of knowledge attracted me to clinical situations where scientific evidence was insufficient and the appropriate course of action was unknown. This interest motivated me to pursue further training in bioethics and to expand my clinical work to palliative medicine and end-of-life care, and I am grateful to Lisa Parker and Bob Arnold for their support in these pursuits. My interest in meaning and limits eventually led me to make a midcareer shift from clinical practice to research. Through the invaluable mentorship of Bill Klein, I was introduced to the theories and methods of decision psychology, which gave me a new way of approaching medical uncertainty. I have since had the good fortune of continuing this research focus, thanks to many opportunities and collaborations with colleagues across the country and around the world.

These colleagues and the ways they have helped me are too numerous to count, but two persons in particular deserve special mention. Ron Epstein not only influenced me through his body of work on mindful practice, but also provided sage guidance on book writing and valuable comments on an earlier draft of the manuscript. He pushed me to sharpen my focus and resist excessive abstraction and intellectualization. His advice improved the manuscript considerably, although I'm afraid I wasn't completely successful in following it.

The colleague to whom I feel most indebted in the writing of this book, however, is the late Renée Fox. It was Renée's pioneering work many years ago that inspired me to make medical uncertainty a focus of my research. I came to know Renée only in the last few years, after she retired from her long and illustrious career. During this time, however, Renée gave me the great gift of her mentorship and friendship. The writing of this book became the impetus for many conversations and visits in which Renée generously shared her wisdom on uncertainty and life in general. She read through drafts of my book and provided not only critical feedback but also the encouragement I needed to move forward. She saw herself, in her own words, as "accompanying" me on a journey, and her companionship helped me cope with my own uncertainty about my work. As fate would have it, Renée died suddenly 2 months ago, and I am filled with feelings of not only sadness and loss, but regret that I did not finish my book in time for her to see the final product. At the same time, I feel deeply grateful for Renée's life and the chance I had to know her and hope at least some of her wisdom and insights will live on through my work.

Yet in both my professional and personal journeys with uncertainty, the most important persons by far have been my family. More than anyone else, my wife, Cindy, has been my constant, loving companion, confidante, and source of strength. Every step of the way—in the writing of this book and in every endeavor of our lives—it has been Cindy's innate hope, optimism, grace, and equanimity that have helped me face the unknown with courage. Our children, Alex, Joey, and Katie, have supported me with their unconditional love, as well as their encouragement and patience through many moments in which I was overly occupied by my work. But they have also inspired me with their sheer creativity, curiosity, and open minds. For Cindy and me, they are the possibilities that keep us moving forward.

Finally, I wish to express my deep gratitude to the Brocher Foundation for hosting me as a Visiting Researcher just before the COVID-19 pandemic broke out. The time I spent there, surrounded by such beauty and tranquility, allowed me to really focus on my writing, think more clearly, and pull this book together. It was a special opportunity in a special place, and I will always be grateful for it.

REFERENCES

Chapter 1

1. Fox RC. *Experiment Perilous: Physicians and Patients Facing the Unknown.* Glencoe, IL: Free Press; 1959.
2. Katz J. *The Silent World of Doctor and Patient.* Vol. *1984.* New York: Free Press; 1984, p. 173.
3. Katz J. Why doctors don't disclose uncertainty. *Hastings Center Report.* 1984;*14*(1):35–44.
4. James W. The will to believe. In *The Will to Believe and Other Essays in Popular Philosophy.* New York: Dover; 1896, p. 13.
5. Nuland S. *The Uncertain Art: Thoughts on a Life in Medicine.* New York: Random House; 2008, p. xv.
6. Fox RC. The evolution of medical uncertainty. *Milbank Memorial Fund Quarterly: Health and Society.* 1980;*58*(1):1–49, p. 34.

Chapter 2

1. James W. The Sentiment of Rationality. In: *The Will to Believe and Other Essays in Popular Philosophy.* Cambridge, MA: Harvard University Press; 1897, pp. 37–57, p. 44.

2. Merriam-Webster Dictionary. *Merriam-Webster Online.*, s.v. "uncertainty." 2010; http://www.merriam-webster.com/uncertainty. Accessed May 1, 2010.

3. *OED Online,* s.v. "Integration." In. *OED Online.* Oxford University Press.

4. Flavell JH. Metacognitive aspects of problem solving. In L. B. Resnick (Ed.), *The nature of intelligence.* Hillsdale: Lawrence Erlbaum; 1979, p. 232, p. 906.

5. Nelson TO. Consciousness and metacognition. *American Psychologist.* 1996;51(2):102–116, p. 104.

6. Smithson M. *Ignorance and Uncertainty: Emerging Paradigms.* New York: Springer Verlag; 1989.

7. Flavell JH. Metacognitive aspects of problem solving. In: Resnick LB, ed. *The Nature of Intelligence.* Hillsdale, N.J.: Erlbaum; 1976:231–236.

8. Miner AC, Reder LM. A new look at feeling of knowing: Its metacognitive role in regulating question answering. In: Metcalfe J, Shimamura AP, eds. *Metacognition: Knowing About Knowing.* Cambridge, MA: MIT Press; 1994:47–70.

9. James W. The Will to Believe. In.: *The Will to Believe and Other Essays in Popular Philosophy.* New York: Dover Publications; 1896, p. 14.

10. Rescher N. *Unknowability: An Inquiry Into the Limits of Knowledge.* Lanham, MD: Lexington Books; 2009.

11. Rescher N. *Ignorance: On the Wider Implications of Deficient Knowledge.* Pittsburgh: University of Pittsburgh Press; 2009.

12. James W. The stream of consciousness (1892). In: Gunn G, ed. *Pragmatism and Other Writings.* New York: Penguin; 2000:171–190, p. 176.

13. Confucius. *The Analects.* London: Penguin UK; 1979, p. 64.

14. Fine G. Does socrates claim to know that he knows nothing? *Oxford Studies in Ancient Philosophy.* 2008;35:49–85.

15. Nelson TO, Narens L. Why investigate metacognition? In: Metcalfe J, Shimamura AP, eds. *Metacognition: Knowing About Knowing.* Cambridge, MA: MIT Press; 1994.

16. Metcalfe J, Shimamura AP, eds. *Metacognition: Knowing About Knowing.* Cambridge, MA: MIT Press; 1994.

17. Schooler JW. Re-representing consciousness: Dissociations between experience and meta-consciousness. *Trends in Cognitive Sciences.* 2002;23:475–483.

18. Efklides A, Papadaki M, Papantoniou G, Kiosseoglou G. Effects of cognitive ability and affect on school mathematics performance and feelings of difficulty. *American Journal of Psychology.* 1997;110:225–258.

19. Efklides A, Papadaki M, Papantoniou G, Kiosseoglou G. Individual differences in school mathematics performance and feelings of difficulty: The effects of cognitive ability, affect, age, and gender. *European Journal of Psychology of Education.* 1999;14:57–69.

20. Dunning D. *Self-insight: Roadblocks and Detours on the Path to Knowing Thyself.* New York: Psychology Press; 2005, p. 12.

21. Dunning D. The Dunning-Kruger effect: On being ignorant of one's own igno-rance. *Advances in Experimental Social Psychology.* 2011;*44*:247–296.

22. Kruger J, Dunning D. Unskilled and unaware of it: How difficulties in recog-nizing one's own incompetence lead to inflated self-assessments. *Journal of Personality and Social Psychology.* 1999;*77* :1121–1134.

23. Rozenblit L, Keil F. The misunderstood limits of folk science: An illusion of explanatory depth. *Cognitive Science.* 2002;*26*:521–562, p. 521, p. 548.

24. Sloman S, Fernbach P. *The Knowledge Illusion: Why We Never Think Alone.* New York: Riverhead Books; 2017.

25. Empiricus S. *Outlines of Scepticism.* Cambridge, UK: Cambridge University Press; 2000, p. 4.

26. Bett R. *Pyrrho, His Antecedents, and His Legacy.* Oxford, UK: Oxford University Press; 2000.

27. Friedman J. Why suspend judging? *Nous.* 2015;*51*:302–326, p. 303, p. 316.

28. Friedman J. Inquiry and belief. *Nous.* 2019;*53*:296–315.

29. Kagan J. *Surprise, Uncertainty, and Mental Structures.* Cambridge, MA: Harvard University Press; 2002.

30. Osman M. An evaluation of dual-process theories of reasoning. *Psychonomic Bulletin and Review.* 2004;*11*:988–1010.

31. Stanovich KE, West RF. On the relative independence of thinking biases and cognitive ability. *Journal of Personality and Social Psychology.* 2008;*94*:672–695.

32. Stanovich KE, West RF. Individual difference in reasoning: Implications for the rationality debate? *Behavioural and Brain Sciences.* 2000;*23*:645–726.

33. Kahneman D. *Thinking, Fast and Slow.* New York: Farrar, Straus, and Giroux; 2011, p. 88.

34. Gilbert DT. How mental systems believe. *American Psychologist.* 1991;*46*:107–119, p. 80.

35. Kleinman A. *Patients and Healers in the Context of Culture.* Berkeley: University of California Press; 1980, p. 105.

36. Charles C, Gafni A, Whelan T. Shared decision-making in the medical encoun-ter: What does it mean? (or it takes at least two to tango). *Social Science and Medicine.* 1997;*44*(5):681–692.

37. Makoul G, Clayman ML. An integrative model of shared decision making in medical encounters. *Patient Education and Counseling.* 2006;*60*(3):301–312.

38. Elwyn G, Durand MA, Song J, et al. A three-talk model for shared decision mak-ing: Multistage consultation process. *British Medical Journal.* 2017;*359*:j4891.

39. Elwyn G, Frosch D, Thomson R, et al. Shared decision making: A model for clinical practice. *Journal of General Internal Medicine.* 2012;*27*(10):1361–1367.

40. Elwyn G, Miron-Shatz T. Deliberation before determination: The definition and evaluation of good decision making. *Health Expectations.* 2010;*13*(2):139–147.

41. Elwyn G, Lloyd A, May C, et al. Collaborative deliberation: A model for patient care. *Patient Education and Counseling.* 2014;*97*(2):158–164.

42. Michaels D, Monforton C. Manufacturing uncertainty: Contested science and the protection of the public's health and environment. *American Journal of Public Health*. 2005;95(Suppl. 1:):S39–S48, p. S39.

43. Pascal B. Pensées. New York: E.P. Dutton; 1958, p. 92, p. 327.

44. Berger PL, Luckmann T. *The Social Construction of Reality: A Treatise in the Sociology of Knowledge*. Garden City, NY: Anchor Books; 1966.

Chapter 3

1. Dewey J. *How We Think*. Boston: D.C. Heath & Co.; 1910, p. 11.

2. Fox RC. Training for Uncertainty. In: Merton R, Reader GC, Kendall P, eds. *The Student-Physician: Introductory Studies in the Sociology of Medical Education*. Cambridge, MA: Harvard University Press; 1957:207–241.

3. Thompson KM. Variability and uncertainty meet risk management and risk communication. *Risk Analysis*. 2002;22(3):647–654.

4. US Environmental Protection Agency. *Guidelines for Carcinogen Risk Assessment*. (Vol EPA/630/P-03/001F:). Washington, DC: U.S. Environmental Protection Agency; 2005.

5. Marks H, Coleman M, Michael M. Further deliberations on uncertainty in risk assessment. *Human and Ecological Risk Assessment*. 2003;9:1399–1410.

6. Apostolakis G. The concept of probability in safety assessments of technological systems. *Science*. 1990;250:1359.

7. Funtowicz SO, Ravetz JR. *Uncertainty and Quality in Science for Policy*. Dordrecht: Kluwer; 1990.

8. Walker WE, Harremoes P. Defining uncertainty: A conceptual basis for uncertainty management in model-based decision support. *Integrated Assessment*. 2003;4(1):5–17.

9. Han PK, Klein WM, Arora NK. Varieties of uncertainty in health care: A conceptual taxonomy. *Medical Decision Making*. 2011;31(6):828–838.

10. *Merriam-Webster Online*, .com. s.v. "Probability."

11. Steyerberg EW. *Clinical Prediction Models: A Practical Approach to Development, Validation, and Updating*. New York: Springer; 2010.

12. Hacking I. *The Taming of Chance*. Cambridge: Cambridge University Press; 1990.

13. Fox CR, Ulkumen G. Distinguishing Two Dimensions of Uncertainty. In: Brun W, Keren G, Kirkebøen G, Montgomery H, eds. *Perspectives on Thinking, Judging, and Decision Making*. Oslo: Universitetsforlaget; 2011.

14. Heisenberg W. *Physics and Philosophy: The Revolution in Modern Science*. New York: Harper; 1958.

15. Smith GD. Epidemiology, epigenetics and the "Gloomy Prospect": Embracing randomness in population health research and practice. *International Journal of Epidemiology.* 2011;40(3):537–562.

16. Johnson C. *Darwin's Dice: The Idea of Chance in the Thought of Charles Darwin.* New York: Oxford University Press; 2015.

17. Tomasetti C, Vogelstein B. Cancer etiology. Variation in cancer risk among tissues can be explained by the number of stem cell divisions. *Science.* 2015;347(6217):78–81.

18. Lindley D. *Uncertainty: Einstein, Heisenberg, Bohr, and the Struggle for the Soul of Science.* New York: Anchor Books; 2008.

19. Cilliers P. *Complexity and Postmodernism.* London: Routledge; 1998.

20. McDaniel RR, Driebe DJ. Uncertainty and Surprise: An Introduction. In: McDaniel RR, Driebe DJ, eds. *Uncertainty and Surprise in Complex Systems.* Berlin: Springer; 2005, pp. 3–11.

21. Reichl LE. Fundamental "Uncertainty" in Science. In: McDaniel RR, Driebe DJ, eds. *Uncertainty and Surprise in Complex Systems.* Berlin: Springer; 2005. pp. 71–76.

22. Boeing G. Visual analysis of nonlinear dynamical systems: Chaos, fractals, self-similarity and the limits of prediction. *Systems.* 2016;4:37.

23. Lorenz EN. Deterministic nonperiodic flow. *Journal of the Atmospheric Sciences.* 1963;20:130–141.

24. Waldrop MW. *Complexity: The Emerging Science at the Edge of Order and Chaos.* New York: Simon and Schuster; 1992.

25. Goldstein J. Emergence as a construct: History and issues. *Emergence—Journal of Complexity Issues in Organizations and Management.* 1999;1:49–72.

26. Knight FH. *Risk, Uncertainty, and Profit.* Boston: Houghton Mifflin; 1921.

27. Ellsberg D. Risk, ambiguity, and the Savage axioms. *Quarterly Journal of Economics.* 1961;75:643–669.

28. Camerer C, Weber M. Recent developments in modeling preferences: Uncertainty and ambiguity. *Journal of Risk and Uncertainty.* 1992;5:325–370.

29. Spiegelhalter DJ, Riesch H. Don't know, can't know: Embracing deeper uncertainties when analysing risks. *Philosophical Transactactions of the Royal Society A: Mathematical, Physical and Engineering Sciences.* 2011;369(1956):4730–4750.

30. Carpenter DM, Geryk LL, Chen AT, Nagler RH, Dieckmann NF, Han PK. Conflicting health information: A critical research need. *Health Expectations.* 2016;19(6):1173–1182.

31. Hacking I. *An Introduction to Probability and Inductive Logic.* New York: Cambridge University Press; 2001, p. 136.

32. Gillies D. *Philosophical Theories of Probability.* London: Routledge; 2000.

33. de Finetti B. *Theory of Probability*. Vol. 1. New York: John Wiley and Sons; 1974, p. 1.

34. Morgan G, Dowlatabadi H, Henrion M, et al., eds. *Best Practice Approaches for Characterizing, Communicating, and Incorporating Scientific Uncertainty in Decisionmaking. A Report by the U.S. Climate Change Science Program and the Subcommittee on Global Change Research (Synthesis and Assessment Product 5.2M)*. Washington, D.C.: National Oceanic and Atmospheric Administration, U.S. Climate Change Science Program; 2009.

35. Han PK. Conceptual, methodological, and ethical problems in communicating uncertainty in clinical evidence. *Medical Care Research and Review*. 20123;72(1, Suppl.):14S–36S.

36. Reyna VF. A theory of medical decision making and health: Fuzzy trace theory. *Medical Decision Making*. 2008;28(6):850–865.

37. Reyna VF, Brainerd CJ. The importance of mathematics in health and human judgment: Numeracy, risk communication, and medical decision making. *Learning and Individual Differences*. 2007;17:147–159.

38. Fox RC. The evolution of medical uncertainty. *Milbank Memorial Fund Quarterly: Health and Society*. 1980;58(1):1–49, p. 34.

39. Hillen MA, Gutheil CM, Strout TD, Smets EM, Han PKJ. Tolerance of uncertainty: Conceptual analysis, integrative model, and implications for healthcare. *Social Science and Medicine*. 2017;180:62–75.

40. Strout TD, Hillen M, Gutheil C, et al. Tolerance of uncertainty: A systematic review of health and healthcare-related outcomes. *Patient Education and Counseling*. 2018;101(9):1518–1537.

Chapter 4

1. Dewey J. *The Quest for Certainty*. Capricorn Books 1960 ed. New York: Capricorn Books, division of G. P. Putnam's Sons; 19291960. First published 1929, p. 227.

2. Rabin M, Thaler RH. Anomalies: Risk aversion. *Journal of Economic Perspectives*. 2001;15:219–232.

3. Weber EU, Blais A, Betz NE. A domain-specific risk-attitude scale: Measuring risk perceptions and risk behaviors. *Journal of Behavioral Decision Making*. 2002;15(4):263–290.

4. Howard RA. The foundations of decision analysis revisited. In: Edwards W, Miles RFJ, Von Winterfeldt D, eds. *Advances in Decision Analysis: From Foundations to Applications*. New York: Cambridge University Press; 2007:32–56.

5. Nau RF. Extensions of the subjective expected utility model. In: Edwards W, Miles RFJ, von Winterfeldt D, eds. *Advances in Decision*

Analysis: From Foundations to Applications. New York: Cambridge University Press; 2007:253–278.

6. Johnson JG, Wilke A, Weber EU. Beyond a trait view of risk taking. *Polish Psychological Bulletin.* 2004;35:153–163.

7. Kahneman D, Tversky A. Prospect theory: An analysis of decision under risk. *Econometrica.* 1979;47:263–291.

8. Slovic P. Perception of risk: Reflections on the psychometric paradigm. In: Krimsky S, Golding D, eds. *Social Theories of Risk.* Westport, CT: Praeger; 1992:117–152.

9. Slovic P. Perception of risk. *Science.* 1987;236:280–285.

10. Anderson EC, Carleton RN, Diefenbach M, Han PKJ. The relationship between uncertainty and affect. *Frontiers in Psychology.* 2019;10:2504.

11. Borkovec TD, Robinson E, Pruzinsky T, DePree JA. Preliminary exploration of worry: Some characteristics and processes. *Behaviour Research and Therapy.* 1983;21:9–16.

12. Robichaud M, Koerner N, Dugas MJ. *Cognitive Behavioral Treatment for Generalized Anxiety Disorder: From Science to Practice.* New York: Routledge; 2019, p. 26.

13. Ellsberg D. Risk, ambiguity, and the Savage axioms. *Quarterly Journal of Economics.* 1961;75:643–669.

14. Arlo-Costa H, Helzner J. Comparative ignorance and the Ellsberg phenomenon. Paper presented at the 4th International Symposium on Imprecise Probabilities and Their Applications; 2005; Pittsburgh, PA; July 2005.

15. Kovařík J, Levin D, Wang T. Ellsberg paradox: Ambiguity and complexity aversions compared. *Journal of Risk and Uncertainty.* 2016;52:47–64.

16. Camerer C, Weber M. Recent developments in modeling preferences: Uncertainty and ambiguity. *Journal of Risk and Uncertainty.* 1992;5:325–370.

17. Einhorn HJ, Hogarth RM. Decision making under ambiguity. *Journal of Business.* 1986;59(4):S225–S250.

18. Einhorn HJ, Hogarth RM. Ambiguity and uncertainty in probabilistic inference. *Psychological Review.* 1985;92(4):433–461.

19. Heath C, Tversky A. Preference and belief: Ambiguity and competence in choice under uncertainty. *Journal of Risk and Uncertainty.* 1991;4:5–28.

20. Kuhn KM. Message format and audience values: Interactive effects of uncertainty information and environmental attitudes on perceived risk. *Journal of Environmental Psychology.* 2000;20:41–51.

21. Winkler RL. Ambiguity, probability, preference, and decision analysis. *Journal of Risk and Uncertainty.* 1991;4:285–297.

22. Lauriola M, Levin IP. Relating individual differences in attitude toward ambiguity to risky choices. *Journal of Behavioral Decision Making.* 2001;14(2):107–122.

23. Han PK, Klein WM, Lehman T, Killam B, Massett H, Freedman AN. Communication of uncertainty regarding individualized cancer risk estimates: Effects and influential factors. *Medical Decision Making.* 2011;*31*(2):354–366.

24. Dieckmann NF, Peters E, Gregory R. At home on the range? Lay interpretations of numerical uncertainty ranges. *Risk Analysis.* 2015;*35*(7): 1281–1295.

25. Viscusi WK. Alarmist decisions with divergent risk information. *The Economic Journal.* 1997;*107*:1657–1670.

26. Viscusi WK, Magat WA, Huber J. Communication of ambiguous risk information. *Theory and Decision.* 1991;*31*:159–173.

27. Viscusi WK, Magat WA, Huber J. Smoking status and public responses to ambiguous scientific risk evidence. *Southern Economic Journal.* 1999;*66*(2):250–270.

28. Han PK, Moser RP, Klein WM. Perceived ambiguity about cancer prevention recommendations: Relationship to perceptions of cancer preventability, risk, and worry. *Journal of Health Communication.* 2006;*11*(Suppl 1):51–69.

29. Carleton RN. Fear of the unknown: One fear to rule them all? *Journal of Anxiety Disorders.* 2016;*41*:5–21, p. 5.

30. Sonsino D, Mandelbaum M. On preference for flexibility and complexity aversion: Experimental evidence. *Theory and Decision.* 2001;*51*:197–216.

31. Buturak G, Evren O. Choice overload and asymmetric regret. *Theoretical Economics.* 2017;*12*:1029–1056.

32. Duttle K, Inukai K. Complexity aversion: Influences of cognitive abilities, culture and system of thought. *Economics Bulletin.* 2015;*35*:846–855.

33. Scheibehenne B, Greifeneder R, Todd PM. Can there ever be too many options? A meta-analytic review of choice overload. *Journal of Consumer Research.* 2010;*37*:409–425.

34. Iyengar SS, Kamenica E. Choice proliferation, simplicity seeking, and asset allocation. *Journal of Public Economics.* 2010;*94*(7):530–539.

35. Iyengar SS, Lepper MR. When choice is demotivating: Can one desire too much of a good thing? *Journal of Personality and Social Psychology.* 2000;*79*:995–1006.

36. Schwartz B. The tyranny of choice. *Scientific American.* 2004;*290*(4):70–75.

37. Speier C, Valacich JS, Vessey I. The influence of task interruption on individual decision making: An information overload perspective. *Decision Sciences.* 1999;*30*:337–360.

38. Redelmeier DA, Shafir E. Medical decision making in situations that offer multiple alternatives. *JAMA.* 1995;*273*(4):302–305.

39. *Merriam-Webster Online.*, s.v. "Regulate." In. *Merriam-Webster.com Dictionary.* https://www.merriam-webster.com/dictionary/regulate. Accessed 6/20/2019.

40. Baumeister RF, Schmeichel BJ, Vohs KD. Self-regulation and the executive function: The self as controlling agent. In: Kruglanski AW, Higgins ET, eds. *Social Psychology: Handbook of Basic Principles* (Seco2nd Edition). New York: Guilford; 2007:516–539.

41. Heatherton TF, Baumeister RF. Self-regulation failure: Past, present, and future. *Psychological Inquiry*. 1996;7:90–98, p. 522.

42. Cole PM, Michel MK, O'Donnell Teti L. The development of emotion regulation and dysregulation: A clinical perspective. *Monographs of the Society for Research in Child Development*. 1994;59:73–100.

43. Gross J. Emotion regulation in adulthood: Timing is everything. *Current Directions in Psychological Science*. 2001;10:214–219.

44. DeSteno D, Gross JJ, Kubzansky L. Affective science and health: The importance of emotion and emotion regulation. *Health Psychology*. 2013;32:474–486.

45. Diefenbach MA, Leventhal H. The common-sense model of illness representation: Theoretical and practical considerations. *Journal of Social Distress and the Homeless*. 1996;5:11–38.

46. Leventhal H, Diefenbach MA, Leventhal EA. Illness cognition: Using common sense to understand treatment adherence and affect cognition interactions. *Cognitive Therapy and Research*. 1992;16:143–163.

47. Han PKJ, Strout TD, Gutheil C, Germann C, King B, Ofstad E, Gulbrandsen P, Trowbridge R. How Physicians Manage Medical Uncertainty: A Qualitative Study and Conceptual Taxonomy. *Med Decis Making*. 2021 Apr;41(3):275–291. doi:10.1177/0272989X21992340. Epub 2021 Feb 15. PMID: 33588616; PMCID: PMC7985858.

48. Robson A, Robinson L. Building on models of information behaviour: Linking information seeking and communication. *Journal of Documentation*. 2013;69:169–193.

49. Claxton K. Bayesian approaches to the value of information: Implications for the regulation of new pharmaceuticals. *Health Economics*. 1999;8(3):269–274.

50. Fenwick E, Claxton K, Sculpher M. The value of implementation and the value of information: Combined and uneven development. *Med Decis Making. Medical Decision Making*.2008;28(1):21–32.

51. Siebert U, Rochau U, Claxton K. When is enough evidence enough?—Using systematic decision analysis and value-of-information analysis to determine the need for further evidence. *Zeitschrift für Evidenz, Fortbildung und Qualität im Gesundheitswesen*. 2013;107(9–10):575–584.

52. Kruglanski AW, Webster DM. Motivated closing of the mind: "Seizing" and "freezing." *Psychological Review*. 1996;103(2):263–283.

53. Sorrentino RM, Roney CJR. *The Uncertain Mind: Individual Differences in Facing the Unknown*. Philadelphia: Taylor & Francis; 2000.

54. Brashers DE. Communication and uncertainty management. *Journal of Communication*. 2001;51:477–497.

55. Babrow AS. Communication and problematic integration: Understanding diverging probability and value, ambiguity, ambivalence, and impossibility. *Communication Theory.* 1992;2(2):95–130.

56. Babrow AS, Kasch CR, Ford LA. The many meanings of uncertainty in illness: Toward a systematic accounting. *Health Communication.* 1998;10(1):1–23.

57. Fox RC. Training for uncertainty. In: Merton R, Reader GC, Kendall P, eds. *The Student-Physician: Introductory Studies in the Sociology of Medical Education.* Cambridge, MA: Harvard University Press; 1957:207–241.

58. James W. The will to believe. In: *The Will to Believe and Other Essays in Popular Philosophy.* New York: Dover Publications; 1896.

59. Neuberg SL, Newsom JT. Personal need for structure: Individual differences in the desire for simple structure. *Journal of Personality and Social Psychology.* 1993;65:113–131.

60. Thompson MM, Naccarato ME, Parker KCH, Moskowitz G. The Personal Need for Structure (PNS) and Personal Fear of Invalidity (PFI) scales: Historical perspectives, present applications and future directions. In: Moskowitz G, ed. *Cognitive Social Psychology: The Princeton Symposium on the Legacy and Future of Social Cognition.* Mahwah, NJ: Erlbaum; 2001:19–39.

61. Bowker GC, Star SL. *Sorting Things Out: Classification and Its Consequences.* Cambridge, MA: MIT Press; 1999, p. 10.

62. Lakoff G. Categories. In: Linguistic Society of Korea, ed. *Linguistics in the Morning Calm: Selected Papers from SICOL-1981* Seoul: Hanshin; 1982, pp. 139–193.

63. James W. Pragmatism. In: Gunn G, ed. *Pragmatism and Other Writings.* New York: Penguin; 1907:1–132, p. 462.

64. Gigerenzer G. *Gut Feelings: The Intelligence of the Unconscious.* New York: Penguin Books; 2007.

65. Simon H. *Models of Man, Social and Rational: Mathematical Essays on Rational Human Behavior in a Social Setting.* New York: Wiley; 1957.

66. Hayes SC. *Rule-Governed Behavior: Cognition, Contingencies, and Instructional Control.* New York: Plenum; 1989.

67. Beauchamp TL, Childress JF. *Principles of Biomedical Ethics.* 8th ed. New York: Oxford University Press; 2013.

68. Empiricus S. *Outlines of Scepticism.* Cambridge, UK: Cambridge University Press; 2000.

69. Bett R. *Pyrrho, His Antecedents, and His Legacy.* Oxford, UK: Oxford University Press; 2000.

70. Williams M. Descartes' transformation of the sceptical tradition. In: Bett R, ed. *The Cambridge Companion to Ancient Scepticism.* Cambridge, UK: Cambridge University Press; 2010:288–313.

71. James W. The sentiment of rationality. In: *The Will to Believe and Other Essays in Popular Philosophy*. Cambridge, MA: Harvard University Press; 1897, pp. 37–57.

72. Elwyn G, Lloyd A, May C, et al. Collaborative deliberation: A model for patient care. *Patient Education and Counseling.* 2014;97(2):158–164.

73. Han PK. Conceptual, methodological, and ethical problems in communicating uncertainty in clinical evidence. *Medical Care Research and Review: MCRR.* 2013;70(1, Suppl.):14S–36S.

74. Han PK. The need for uncertainty: a case for prognostic silence. *Perspectives in Biology and Medicine.* 2016;59(4):567–575.

75. Innes S, Payne S. Advanced cancer patients' prognostic information preferences: A review. *Palliative Medicine.* 2009;23(1):29–39.

76. Helft PR. An intimate collaboration: prognostic communication with advanced cancer patients. *Journal of Clinical Ethics.* 2006;17(2):110–121.

77. Christakis NA. *Death Foretold: Prophecy and Prognosis in Medical Care.* Chicago: University of Chicago; 1999.

78. Han PKJ, Gutheil C, Hutchinson RN, LaChance JA. Cause or Effect? The Role of Prognostic Uncertainty in the Fear of Cancer Recurrence. *Front Psychol.* 2021 Jan 15;11:626038. doi:10.3389/fpsyg.2020.626038. PMID: 33519656; PMCID: PMC7843433.

79. Ong AD, Bergeman CS, Bisconti TL, Wallace KA. Psychological resilience, positive emotions, and successful adaptation to stress in later life. *Journal of Personality and Social Psychology.* 2006;91:730–749.

80. Merluzzi TV, Errol PJ. "Letting go": From ancient to modern perspectives on relinquishing personal control—A theoretical perspective on religion and coping with cancer. *Journal of Religion and Health.* 2017;56:2039–2052.

81. Sellars J. *Stoicism.* Berkeley: University of California Press; 2006.

82. de Finetti B. *Theory of Probability.* Vol. 1. New York: John Wiley and Sons; 1974.

83. Suls J, Fletcher B. The relative efficacy of avoidant and nonavoidant coping strategies: A meta-analysis. *Health Psychology.* 1985;4:249–288.

84. Skinner EA, Edge K, Altman J. Searching for the structure of coping: A review and critique of category systems for classifying ways of coping. *Psychological Bulletin.* 2003;129:216–269.

85. Carver CS, Scheier MF, Weintraub JK. Assessing coping strategies: A theoretically based approach. *Journal of Personality and Social Psychology. J Pers Soc Psychol.* 1989;56:267–283.

86. Lazarus RS. Coping theory and research: Past, present, and future. *Psychosomatic Medicine.* 1993;55:234–247.

87. Lazarus RS, Folkman S. *Stress, Appraisal, and Coping.* New York: Springer; 1984.

88. Robichaud M. Cognitive behavior therapy targeting intolerance of uncertainty: application to a clinical case of generalized anxiety disorder. *Cognitive and Behavioral Practice.* 2013;20:251–263.

89. Carleton RN. The intolerance of uncertainty construct in the context of anxiety disorders: Theoretical and practical perspectives. *Expert Review of Neurotherapeutics.* 2012;12(8):937–947.

90. Fox RC. *Experiment Perilous: Physicians and Patients Facing the Unknown.* Glencoe, IL: Free Press; 1959.

91. Rasmussen HN, Wrosch C, Scheier M, Carver CS. Self-regulation processes and health: The importance of optimism and goal adjustment. *Journal of Personality.* 2006;74:1721–1748.

92. Carver CS, Scheier M. Self-regulation and its failures. *Psychological Inquiry.* 1996;7:32–40.

93. Steele CM. The psychology of self-affirmation: Sustaining the integrity of the self. *Advances in Experimental Social Psychology.* 1988;21:261–302.

94. Harris PR, Epton T. The impact of self-affirmation on health cognition, health behavior, and other health-related responses: A narrative review. *Social and Personality Psychology Compass.* 2009;3:962–978.

95. McQueen A, Klein WMP. Experimental manipulations of self-affirmation: A systematic review. *Self and Identity.* 2006;5:289–354.

96. Klein WMP, Harris PR, Ferrer RA, Zajac LE. Feelings of vulnerability in response to threatening messages: Effects of self-affirmation. *Journal of Experimental Social Psychology.* 2011;47:1237–1242.

97. Gable SL, Reis HT, Impett EA, Asher ER. What do you do when things go right? The intrapersonal and interpersonal benefits of sharing positive events. *Journal of Personality and Social Psychology.* 2004;87:228–245.

98. Lambert NM, Gwinn AM, Baumeister RF, et al. The perks of sharing positive experiences and grateful experiences. *Journal of Social & Personal Relationships.* 2013;30:24–43.

99. Pennebaker JW, Zech E, Rimé B. Disclosing and sharing emotion: Psychological, social and health consequences. In: M.S. Stroebe WMS, R.O. Hansson RO, Stroebe W, & H. Schut H, ed. *Handbook of Bereavement Research: Consequences, Coping, and Care.* Washington DC: American Psychological Association; 2001:517–539.

100. Kennedy-Moore E, Watson JC. How and when does emotional expression help? *Review of General Psychology.* 2001;5:187–212.

101. Rossignac-Milon M, Higgins ET. Epistemic companions: Shared reality development in close relationships. *Current Opinion in Psychology.* 2018;23:66–71, p. 66, p. 67.

102. Pinel E. Existential isolation and I-sharing: Interpersonal and intergroup implications. *Current Opinion in Psychology.* 2018;23:84–87.

103. Wagner U, Galli L, Schott BH, et al. Beautiful friendship: Social sharing of emotions improves subjective feelings and activates the neural reward circuitry. *Social Cognitive and Affective Neuroscience.* 2015;10:801–808.

104. Kleinman, A. *The Soul of Care: The Moral Education of a Husband and a Doctor.* New York: Viking. 2019, p. 249.

105. Mishel MH. Uncertainty in illness. *Image— The Journal of Nursing Scholarship.* 1988;*20*(4):225–232.

106. Mishel MH. Reconceptualization of the uncertainty in illness theory. *Image— The Journal of Nursing Scholarship J Nurs Sch.* 1990;22(4):256–262.

Chapter 5

1. Groopman JE. *How Doctors Think.* New York: Houghton Mifflin; 2007, p. 4.

2. Rasmussen HN, Wrosch C, Scheier M, Carver CS. Self-regulation processes and health: The importance of optimism and goal adjustment. *Journal of Personality.* 2006;74:1721–1748.

3. Carver CS, Scheier M. Self-regulation and its failures. *Psychological Inquiry.* 1996;7:32–40.

4. Frenkel-Brunswik E. Intolerance of ambiguity as an emotional and perceptual personality variable. *Journal of Personality.* 1949;*18*.

5. Hillen MA, Gutheil CM, Strout TD, Smets EM, Han PKJ. Tolerance of uncertainty: Conceptual analysis, integrative model, and implications for healthcare. *Social Science and Medicine.* 2017;*180*:62–75.

6. Carleton RN. The intolerance of uncertainty construct in the context of anxiety disorders: Theoretical and practical perspectives. *Expert Review of Neurotherapeutics.* 2012;*12*(8):937–947.

7. Carleton RN. Fear of the unknown: One fear to rule them all? *Journal of Anxiety Disorders.* 2016;*41*:5–21, p. 5.

8. Koerner N, Dugas MJ. An investigation of appraisals in individuals vulnerable to excessive worry: The role of intolerance of uncertainty. *Cognitive Therapy and Research.* 2008;32:619–638.

9. Borkovec TD, Robinson E, Pruzinsky T, DePree JA. Preliminary exploration of worry: Some characteristics and processes. *Behaviour Research and Therapy.* 1983;*21*:9–16.

10. Ladouceur R, Talbot F, Dugas MJ. Behavioral expressions of intolerance of uncertainty in worry. Experimental findings. *Behavior Modification.* 1997;*21*(3):355–371.

11. Shihata S, McEvoy PM, Mullan BA, Carleton RN. Intolerance of uncertainty in emotional disorders: What uncertainties remain? *Journal of Anxiety Disorders.* 2016;*41*:115–124.

12. Robichaud M, Koerner N, Dugas MJ. *Cognitive Behavioral Treatment for Generalized Anxiety Disorder: From Science to Practice.* New York: Routledge; 2019.

13. Boelen PA, Carleton RN. Intolerance of uncertainty, hypochondriacal concerns, obsessive-compulsive symptoms, and worry. *The Journal of Nervous and Mental Disease*. 2012;200(3):208–213.

14. Fox RC. Training for uncertainty. In: Merton R, Reader GC, Kendall P, eds. *The Student-Physician: Introductory Studies in the Sociology of Medical Education*. Cambridge, MA: Harvard University Press; 1957:207–241.

15. Fox RC. *Experiment Perilous: Physicians and Patients Facing the Unknown*. Glencoe, IL: Free Press; 1959.

16. Back AL, Arnold RM, Quill TE. Hope for the best, and prepare for the worst. *Annals of Internal Medicine*. 2003;138(5):439–443.

17. Kleinman A. *What Really Matters: Living a Moral Life Amidst Uncertainty and Danger*. New York: Oxford University Press; 2007, pp. 234–235.

18. Paine DR, Sandage SJ, Rupert D, Devor NG, Bronstein M. Humility as a psychotherapeutic virtue: Spiritual, philosophical, and psychological foundations. *Journal of Spirituality in Mental Health*. 2015;17:3–25.

19. Tangney JP. Humility: Theoretical perspectives, empirical findings and directions for future research. *Journal of Social and Clinical Psychology*. 2000;19:70–82.

20. Whitcomb D, Battaly H, Baehr J, Howard-Snyder D. Intellectual humility: Owning our limitations. *Philosophy and Phenomenological Research*. 2015;91:1–31.

21. Hazlett A. Higher-order epistemic attitudes and intellectual humility. *Episteme*. 2012;9:205–223, p. 206.

22. Leary MR, Diebels KJ, Davisson EK, et al. Cognitive and interpersonal features of intellectual humility. *Personality and Social Psychology Bulletin*. 2017;43:793–813.

23. Deffler SA, Leary MR, Hoyle RH. Knowing what you know: Intellectual humility and judgments of recognition memory. *Personality and Individual Differences*. 2016;96 :255–259.

24. Krumrei-Mancuso EJ, Rouse SV. The development and validation of the comprehensive Intellectual Humility Scale. *Journal of Personality Assessment*. 2016;98 :209–221.

25. Hayes SC, Luoma JB, Bond FW, Masuda A, Lillis J. Acceptance and commitment therapy: Model, processes and outcomes. *Behavior Research and Therapy*. 2006;44:1–25, p. 7.

26. Kashdan TB, Rottenberg J. Psychological flexibility as a fundamental aspect of health. *Clinical Psychology Review*. 2010;30:865–878, p. 866, p. 876.

27. Rachman SJ. Fear and courage: A psychological perspective. *Social Research*. 2004;71:149–176, p. 173.

28. Woodard C, Pury C. The construct of courage: Categorization and measurement. *Consulting Psychology Journal: Practice and Research*. 2004;59(2):135–147, p. 136.

29. Tillich P. *The Courage to Be*. New Haven: Yale University Press; 1952, p. 86.
30. May R. *Man's Search for Himself*. New York: W.W. Norton & Company; 1953, p. 179.
31. Dewey J. *How We Think*. Boston: D.C. Heath & Co.; 1910.
32. Paul C. The relentless therapeutic imperative. *BMJ*. 2004;329(7480): 1457–1459.
33. Han PK. The need for uncertainty: A case for prognostic silence. *Perspectives in Biology and Medicine*. 2016;59(4):567–575.
34. Helft PR. Necessary collusion: Prognostic communication with advanced cancer patients. *Journal of Clinical Oncology*. 2005;23(13):3146–3150.
35. Helft PR. An intimate collaboration: Prognostic communication with advanced cancer patients. *Journal of Clinical Ethics*. 2006;17(2):110–121.
36. Han PKJ, Gutheil C, Hutchinson RM, Lachance JA. Cause or effect? The role of prognostic uncertainty in the fear of cancer recurrence. *Front Psychol*. 2021 Jan 15;11:626038. doi:10.3389/fpsyg.2020.626038. PMID: 33519656; PMCID: PMC7843433.

Chapter 6

1. Katz, J. *The Silent World of Doctor and Patient*. Baltimore: Johns Hopkins University Press. 1984, p. 206, p. xv.
2. Katz J. *The Silent World of Doctor and Patient*. Vol. *1984*. New York: Free Press; 1984.
3. Engelhardt EG, Pieterse AH, Han PK, et al. Disclosing the uncertainty associated with prognostic estimates in breast cancer. *Medical Decision Making*. 2017;37(3):179–192.
4. Elwyn G, Miron-Shatz T. Deliberation before determination: The definition and evaluation of good decision making. *Health Expectations*. 2010;13(2):139–147.
5. Elwyn G, Frosch D, Thomson R, et al. Shared decision making: A model for clinical practice. *Journal of General Internal Medicine*. 2012;27(10):1361–1367.
6. Elwyn G, Durand MA, Song J, et al. A three-talk model for shared decision making: Multistage consultation process. *BMJ*. 2017;359:j4891.
7. Liu BF, Bartz L, Duke N. Communicating crisis uncertainty: a review of the knowledge gaps. *Public Relations Review*. 2016;42:479–487.
8. Seeger MW. Best practices in crisis communication: An expert panel process. *Journal of Applied Communication Research*. 2006;34(3):232–244.
9. Berg JW. All for one and one for all: Informed consent and public health. *Houston Law Review*. 2012;50 Hou. L. Rev. 1.
10. Covello VT. Best practices in public health risk and crisis communication. *Journal of Health Communication*. 2003;8(Suppl. 1):5–8; discussion 148–151.

11. National Academies of Sciences, Engineering, and Medicine. *Communicating Science Effectively: A Research Agenda.* In. Washington, DC: The National Academies Press; 2017.

12. Ancker JS, Senathirajah Y, Kukafka R, Starren JB. Design features of graphs in health risk communication: A systematic review. *Journal of the American Medical Informatics Association.* 2006;*13*(6):608–618.

13. Lipkus IM. Numeric, verbal, and visual formats of conveying health risks: suggested best practices and future recommendations. *Medical Decision Making.* 2007;*27*(5):696–713.

14. Lipkus IM, Hollands JG. The visual communication of risk. *Journal of the National Cancer Institute Monographs.* 1999(;(25):149–163.

15. Spiegelhalter D, Pearson M, Short I. Visualizing uncertainty about the future. *Science.* 2011;*333*(6048):1393–1400.

16. Gigerenzer G, Gaissmaier W, Kurz-Milcke E, Schwartz LM, Woloshin S. Helping doctors and patients make sense of health statistics. *Psychological Science in the Public Interest.* 2007;*8*:53–96.

17. Kurz-Milcke E, Gigerenzer G, Martignon L. Transparency in risk communication: Graphical and analog tools. *Annals of the New York Academy of Sciences.* 2008;*1128*:18–28.

18. Bansback N, Bell M, Spooner L, Pompeo A, Han PKJ, Harrison M. Communicating uncertainty in benefits and harms: A review of patient decision support interventions. *Patient.* 2017;*10*(3):311–319.

19. Harrison M, Han PKJ, Rabin B, et al. Communicating uncertainty in cancer prognosis: A review of web-based prognostic tools. *Patient Education and Counseling.* 20182019;*102*(5):842–849.

20. Han PK. Conceptual, methodological, and ethical problems in communicating uncertainty in clinical evidence. *Medical Care Research Review.* 2013;*70*(1, Suppl.):14S–36S.

21. Engelhardt EG, Pieterse AH, Han PK, van Duijn-Bakker N, Cluitmans F, Maartense E, Bos MM, Weijl NI, Punt CJ, Quarles van Ufford-Mannesse P, Sleeboom H, Portielje JE, van der Hoeven KJ, Woei-A-Jin FJ, Kroep JR, de Haes HC, Smets EM, Stiggelbout AM. Disclosing the uncertainty associated with prognostic estimates in breast cancer. *Med Decis Making.* 2017 Apr;*37*(3):179–192.

22. Balshem H, Helfand M, Schunemann HJ, et al. GRADE guidelines: 3. Rating the quality of evidence. *Journal of Clinical Epidemiology.* 2011;*64*(4):401–406.

23. Guyatt G, Oxman AD, Akl EA, et al. GRADE guidelines: 1. Introduction—GRADE evidence profiles and summary of findings tables. *Journal of Clinical Epidemiology.* 2011;*64*(4):383–394.

24. Guyatt GH, Oxman AD, Vist GE, et al. GRADE: An emerging consensus on rating quality of evidence and strength of recommendations. *BMJ.* 2008;*336*(7650):924–926.

25. Hacking I. *An Introduction to Probability and Inductive Logic.* New York: Cambridge University Press; 2001.

26. Hacking I. *The Emergence of Probability.* Cambridge: Cambridge University Press; 1975.

27. Reyna VF. A theory of medical decision making and health: Fuzzy trace theory. *Medical Decision Making.* 2008;28(6):850–865.

28. Reyna VF, Brainerd CJ. Dual processes in decision making and developmental neuroscience: A fuzzy-trace model. *Developmental Review.* 2011;31(2–3):180–206.

29. Reyna VF, Nelson WL, Han PK, Dieckmann NF. How numeracy influences risk comprehension and medical decision making. *Psychological Bulletin.* 2009;135(6):943–973.

30. Zikmund-Fisher BJ. The right tool is what they need, not what we have: A taxonomy of appropriate levels of precision in patient risk communication. *Medical Care Research and Review.* 20132;70(1, Suppl.):37S–49S.

31. Han PK, Joekes K, Elwyn G, et al. Development and evaluation of a risk communication curriculum for medical students. *Patient Education and Counseling.* 2013;94(1):43–49.

32. Legare F, Moumjid-Ferdjaoui N, Drolet R, et al. Core competencies for shared decision making training programs: Insights from an international, interdisciplinary working group. *The Journal of Continuing Education in the Health Professions.* 2013;33(4):267–273.

33. Legare F, Politi MC, Drolet R, et al. Training health professionals in shared decision-making: An international environmental scan. *Patient Education and Counseling.* 2012;88(2):159–169.

34. US Centers for Disease Control and Prevention. *CERC Manual: 2018 Update. Crisis & Emergency Risk Communication (CERC).* 2018. https://emergency.cdc.gov/cerc/manual/index.asp.

35. Hofer BK. Personal epistemology research: Implications for learning and teaching. *J Educational Psychology Review.* 2001;13(4):353–383.

36. Hofer BK, Pintrich PR, eds. *Personal Epistemology: The Psychology of Beliefs About Knowledge and Knowing.* New York: Routledge; 2002.

37. Pintrich PR. Future challenges and directions for theory and research on personal epistemology. In: Hofer BK, Pintrich PR, eds. *Personal Epistemology: The Psychology of Beliefs About Knowledge and Knowing.* New York: Routledge; 2002:389–414.

38. Schommer-Atkins M. An evolving theoretical framework for an epistemological belief system. In: Hofer BK, Pintrich PR, eds. *Personal Epistemology: The Psychology of Beliefs About Knowledge and Knowing.* New York: Routledge; 2002:103–118.

39. Rule DC, Bendixen LD. The integrative model of personal epistemology development: Theoretical underpinnings and implications for education. In:

Bendixen LD, Feucht FC, eds. *Personal Epistemology in the Classroom: Theory, Research, and Implications for Practice.* Cambridge: Cambridge University Press; 2010:94–123.

40. Perry WG. *Forms of Intellectual and Ethical Development in the College Years.* New York: Holt, Rinehart, and Winston; 1970.

41. Kienhues D, Bromme R, Stahl E. Changing epistemological beliefs: The unexpected impact of a short-term intervention. *The British Journal of Educational Psychology.* 2008;78(Pt. 4):545–565.

42. Trautwein U, Lüdtke O. Epistemological beliefs, school achievement, and college major: A large-scale longitudinal study on the impact of certainty beliefs. *Contemporary Educational Psychology.* 2007;32:348–366.

43. King PM, Kitchener KS. The reflective judgment model: Twenty years of research on epistemic cognition. In: Hofer BK, Pintrich PR, eds. *Personal Epistemology: The Psychology of Beliefs About Knowledge and Knowing.* New York: Routledge; 2002:37–61.

44. King PM, Kitchener KS. *Developing Reflective Judgment: Understanding and Promoting Intellectual Growth and Critical Thinking in Adolescents and Adults.* San Francisco: Jossey-Bass; 1994.

45. Winkler RL. Ambiguity, probability, preference, and decision analysis. *Journal of Risk and Uncertainty.* 1991;4:285–297.

46. Chow CC, Sarin RK. Known, unknown, and unknowable uncertainties. *Theory and Decision.* 2002;52:127–138.

47. Han PKJ, Scharnetzki E, Scherer AM, Thorpe A, Lary C, Waterston L, Fagerlin A, Dieckmann N. Communicating scientific uncertainty about the COVID-19 pandemic: Beneficial effects of an uncertainty-normalizing strategy. *J Med Internet Res.* 2021 Mar 21. doi:10.2196/27832. Epub ahead of print. PMID: 33769947.

48. Fox RC. The evolution of medical uncertainty. *Milbank Memorial Fund Quarterly: Health and Society.* 1980;58(1):1–49, p. 7.

49. Fox RC. Training for Uncertainty. In: Merton R, Reader GC, Kendall P, eds. *The Student-Physician: Introductory Studies in the Sociology of Medical Education.* Cambridge, MA: Harvard University Press; 1957:207–241.

50. Fox RC. *Experiment Perilous: Physicians and Patients Facing the Unknown.* Glencoe, IL: Free Press; 1959.

51. Gowda D, Dubroff R, Willieme A, Swan-Sein A, Capello C. Art as sanctuary: A four-year mixed-methods evaluation of a visual art course addressing uncertainty through reflection. *Academic Medicine.* 2018;93(11S Association of American Medical Colleges Learn Serve Lead: Proceedings of the 57th Annual Research in Medical Education Sessions):S8–S13.

52. Hailey D, Miller AM, Yenawine P. Understanding visual literacy: The visual thinking strategies approach. In: Baylen DM, D'Alba A, eds. *Essentials of*

Teaching and Integrating Visual and Media Literacy. Switzerland: Springer; 2015, pp. 49–73.

53. Bentwich ME, Gilbey P. More than visual literacy: Art and the enhancement of tolerance for ambiguity and empathy. *BMC Medical Education.* 2017;*17*(1):200.

54. Watson K, Fu B. Medical improv: A novel approach to teaching communication and professionalism skills. *Annals of Internal Medicine.* 2016;*165*(8):591–592.

55. Shochet R, King J, Levine R, Clever S, Wright S. "Thinking on my feet": An improvisation course to enhance students' confidence and responsiveness in the medical interview. *Education for Primary Care.* 2013;*24*(2):119–124.

56. Ofri D. Medical humanities: The Rx for uncertainty? *Academic Medicine.* 2017;*92*(12):1657–1658, p. 1658.

57. Tonelli MR, Upshur REG. A philosophical approach to addressing uncertainty in medical education. *Academic Medicine.* 2019;*94*(4):507–511.

58. Witte CL, Witte MH, Kerwin A. Ignorance and the process of learning and discovery in medicine. *Controlled Clinical Trials.* 1994;*15*(1):1–4, p. 25.

59. Witte MH, Kerwin A, Witte CL, Scadron A. A curriculum on medical ignorance. *Medical Education.* 1989;*23*(1):24–29.

60. Cassel CK, Guest JA. Choosing wisely: Helping physicians and patients make smart decisions about their care. *JAMA.* 2012;*307*(17):1801–1802.

61. Welch G, Schwartz LM, Woloshin S. *Overdiagnosed: Making People Sick in Pursuit of Health.* Boston: Beacon Press; 2011.

62. Brownlee S. *Overtreated: Why Too Much Medicine Is Making Us Sicker and Poorer.* New York: Bloomsbury; 2007.

63. Knorr Cetina K. *Epistemic Cultures: How the Sciences Make Knowledge.* Cambridge, MA: Harvard University Press; 1999.

64. Academy of Medical Royal Colleges (AoMRC). *Reflective Practice Toolkit.* 2018. http://www.aomrc.org.uk/wp-content/uploads/2018/08/Reflective_Practice_Toolkit_AoMRC_CoPMED_0818.pdf. Accessed November 9, 2019, p. 1.

65. Schon D. *The Reflective Practitioner: How Professionals Think in Action.* New York: Basic Books; 1983, p. 268.

66. Epstein RM. Mindful practice. *JAMA.* 1999;*282*(9):833–839, p. 835.

67. Epstein RM, Siegel DJ, Silberman J. Self-monitoring in clinical practice: A challenge for medical educators. *The Journal of Continuing Education in the Health Professions.* 2008;*28*(1):5–13, p. 7.

68. Epstein R. *Attending: Medicine, Mindfulness, and Humanity.* New York: Scribner; 2017, p. 57, p. 65.

69. Epstein RM. Reflection, perception and the acquisition of wisdom. *Medical Education.* 2008;*42*(11):1048–1050.

70. Krasner MS, Epstein RM, Beckman H, et al. Association of an educational program in mindful communication with burnout, empathy, and attitudes among primary care physicians. *JAMA.* 2009;*302*(12):1284–1293.

71. Danczak A, Lea A. Developing expertise for uncertainty; do we rely on a baptism of fire, the mills of experience or could clinicians be trained? *Education for Primary Care.* 2018;*29*(4):237–241.

72. George RE, Lowe WA. Well-being and uncertainty in health care practice. *Clinical Teacher.* 2019;*16*(4):298–305.

73. Grant A, McKimm J, Murphy F. *Developing Reflective Practice: A Guide for Medical Students, Doctors, and Teachers.* Chichester, UK: Wiley Blackwell.

74. Hollnagel E, Braithwaite J, Wears RL. Preface: On the need for resilience in health care. In: Hollnagel E, Braithwaite J, Wears RL, eds. *Resilient Health Care.* Dorchester, UK: Ashgate; 2015:xix–xxvi, p. xxv.

75. Cook R. Resilience, the Second Story, and Progress on Patient Safety. In: Hollnagel E, Braithwaite J, Sears RL, eds. *Resilient Health Care.* Dorchester, UK: Ashgate; 2015:19–26.

76. Nyssen AS, Blavier A. Investigating expertise, flexibility and resilience in socio-technical environments: A case study in robotic surgery. In: Hollnagel E, Braithwaite J, Sears RL, eds. *Resilient Health Care.* Dorchester, UK: Ashgate; 2015:97–110, p. 98.

77. Sheps S, Cardiff K. Resilient health care. In: Hollnagel E, Braithwaite J, Sears RL, eds. *Resilient Health Care.* Dorchester, UK: Ashgate; 2015:49–56.

78. Plsek PE, Greenhalgh T. Complexity science: The challenge of complexity in health care. *BMJ.* 2001;*323*(7313):625–628.

79. Greenhalgh T, Papoutsi C. Studying complexity in health services research: Desperately seeking an overdue paradigm shift. *BMC Medicine.* 2018;*16*(1):95, p. 2.

80. Hollnagel E. Making health care resilient: From safety-I to safety-II. In: Hollnagel E, Braithwaite J, Sears RL, eds. *Resilient Health Care.* Dorchester, UK: Ashgate; 2015:3–18.

81. Clay-Williams R, Braithwaite J. Safety-II thinking in action: " 'Just in Time' " information to support everyday activities. In: Hollnagel E, Braithwaite J, Sears RL, eds. *Resilient Health Care.* Dorchester, UK: Ashgate; 2015:205–214.

82. Sutcliffe KM, Weick KE. Mindful organising and resilient health care. In: Hollnagel E, Braithwaite J, Sears RL, eds. *Resilient Health Care.* Dorchester, UK: Ashgate; 2015:145–158, p. 149.

83. Braithwaite J, Clay-Williams R, Nugus P, Plumb J. Health care as a complex adaptive system. *In:* Hollnagel E, Braithwaite J, Sears RL, eds. *Resilient Health Care.* Dorchester, UK: Ashgate; 2015:57–76, p. 58.

84. Hollnagel E, Braithwaite J, Sears RL. Epilogue: How to make health care resilient. In: Hollnagel E, Braithwaite J, Sears RL, eds. *Resilient Health Care.* Dorchester, UK: Ashgate; 2015:227–238, p. 230.

85. McDaniel RR, Driebe DJ. Uncertainty and surprise: An introduction. In: McDaniel RR, Driebe DJ, eds. *Uncertainty and Surprise in Complex Systems*. Berlin: Springer; 2005:3–11, p. 8.

86. Robichaud M, Koerner N, Dugas MJ. *Cognitive Behavioral Treatment for Generalized Anxiety Disorder: From Science to Practice*. New York: Routledge; 2019, p. 84.

87. Boswell JF, Thompson-Hollands J, Farchione TJ, Barlow DH. Intolerance of uncertainty: A common factor in the treatment of emotional disorders. *Journal of Clinical Psychology*. 2013;69(6):630–645.

88. Carleton RN. The intolerance of uncertainty construct in the context of anxiety disorders: Theoretical and practical perspectives. *Expert Review of Neurotherapeutics*. 2012;12(8):937–947.

89. Robichaud M. Cognitive behavior therapy targeting intolerance of uncertainty: Application to a clinical case of generalized anxiety disorder. *Cognitive and Behavioral Practice*. 2013;20 :251–263.

90. Boelen PA, Carleton RN. Intolerance of uncertainty, hypochondriacal concerns, obsessive-compulsive symptoms, and worry. *The Journal of Nervous and Mental Disease*. 2012;200(3):208–213.

91. Carleton RN. Into the unknown: A review and synthesis of contemporary models involving uncertainty. *Journal of Anxiety Disorders*. 2016;39:30–43.

92. Carleton RN, Mulvogue MK, Thibodeau MA, McCabe RE, Antony MM, Asmundson GJ. Increasingly certain about uncertainty: Intolerance of uncertainty across anxiety and depression. *Journal of Anxiety Disorders*. 2012;26(3):468–479.

93. Buhr K, Dugas M. Intolerance for uncertainty scale: Psychometric properties of the English version. *Behaviour Research and Therapy*. 2002;40:931–946.

94. Buhr K, Dugas MJ. The role of fear of anxiety and intolerance of uncertainty in worry: an experimental manipulation. *Behaviour Research and Therapy*. 2009;47(3):215–223.

95. Robichaud M, Dugas MJ. *The Generalized Anxiety Disorder Workbook: A Comprehensive CBT Guide for Coping With Uncertainty, Worry, and Fear*. Oakland, CA: New Harbinger Publications, Inc.; 2015.

96. Wells A. Metacognitive theory and therapy for worry and generalized anxiety disorder: Review and status. *Journal of Experimental Psychopathology*. 2010;1:133–145, p. 140.

97. Hayes SC, Luoma JB, Bond FW, Masuda A, Lillis J. Acceptance and commitment therapy: Model, processes and outcomes. *Behaviour Research and Therapy*. 2006;44:1–25.

98. Chin F, Hayes SC. Acceptance and commitment therapy and the cognitive behavioral tradition: Assumptions, model, methods, and outcomes. In: Hofmann SG, Asmundson GJ, eds. *The Science of Cognitive Behavioral Therapy*. Amsterdam: Elsevier; 2017:155–173, p. 161.

99. Cooper M. *Existential Therapies*. 2nd ed. Thousand Oaks, CA: Sage; 2016.

100. Yalom I. *Existential Psychotherapy*. New York: Basic Books; 1980.

101. Frankl V. *The Will to Meaning: Foundations and Applications of Logotherapy*. New York: Plume; 1970.

102. Tillich P. *Dynamics of Faith*. New York: Harper & Row; 1957.

103. May R. *Man's Search for Himself*. New York: W.W. Norton & Company; 1953.

104. Breitbart WS, Poppito SR. *Individual Meaning-Centered Psychotherapy for Patients with Advanced Cancer*. New York: Oxford University Press; 2014.

105. Mishel MH, Germino BB, Gil KM, et al. Benefits from an uncertainty management intervention for African-American and Caucasian older long-term breast cancer survivors. *Psychooncology*. 2005;14(11):962–978.

106. Chochinov HM, Hack T, Hassard T, Kristjanson LJ, McClement S, Harlos M. Dignity therapy: A novel psychotherapeutic intervention for patients near the end of life. *Journal of Clinical Oncology*. 2005;23(24):5520–5525.

107. Chochinov HM, Kristjanson LJ, Breitbart W, et al. Effect of dignity therapy on distress and end-of-life experience in terminally ill patients: A randomised controlled trial. *Lancet Oncology*. 2011;12(8):753–762.

108. Smith SM, Cousins G, Clyne B, Allwright S, O'Dowd T. Shared care across the interface between primary and specialty care in management of long term conditions. *Cochrane Database Systematic Reviews*. 2017;2(2):CD004910.

109. Hickman M, Drummond N, Grimshaw J. A taxonomy of shared care for chronic disease. *Journal of Public Health Medicine*. 1994;16(4):447–454.

110. American Psychiatric Association, Academy of Psychosomatic Medicine. Report on Dissemination of Integrated Care: *Dissemination of Integrated Care Within Adult Primary Care Settings: The Collaborative Care Model*. 2016. https://www.psychiatry.org/psychiatrists/practice/professional-interests/integrated-care/learn. Accessed March 8, 2020.

111. Gittell JH. Coordinating mechanisms in care provider groups: Relational coordination as a mediator and input uncertainty as a moderator of performance effects. *Management Science*. 2002;48:1408–1426, p. 210.

112. Gittell JH, Godfrey M, Thistlethwaite J. Interprofessional collaborative practice and relational coordination: improving healthcare through relationships. *Journal of Interprofessional Care*. 2013;27(3):210–213.

113. Han PKJ, Babrow A, Hillen MA, Gulbrandsen P, Smets EM, Ofstad EH. Uncertainty in health care: Towards a more systematic program of research. *Patient Education and Counseling*. 2019 Oct;102(10):1756–1766.

114. Epstein RM, Street RL, Jr. Shared mind: Communication, decision making, and autonomy in serious illness. *Annals of Family Medicine*. 2011;9(5):454–461, p. 454, p. 457.

115. Rossignac-Milon M, Higgins ET. Epistemic companions: Shared reality development in close relationships. *Current Opinion in Psychology*. 2018;23:66–71.

116. Pinel E. Existential isolation and I-sharing: Interpersonal and intergroup implications. *Current Opinion in Psychology.* 2018;23:84–87.

117. US Department of Veterans Affairs. *Whole Health.* https://www.va.gov/WHOLEHEALTH/index.asp. 2020. Accessed November 1, 2020, 2020.

118. James W. Is life worth living? 1897. In: Gunn G, ed. *Pragmatism and Other Writings.* New York: Penguin; 2000:219–241, p. 238.

119. James W. The dilemma of determinism. In: McDermott JJ, ed. *The Writings of William James.* Chicago: University of Chicago; 1967:587–610, p. 77, p. 89.

120. James W. Pragmatism. 1907. In: Gunn G, ed. *Pragmatism and Other Writings.* New York: Penguin; 2000:1–132, p. 28, p. 29, p. 112.

121. James W. The will to believe. 1897. In: Gunn G, ed. *Pragmatism and Other Writings.* New York: Penguin; 2000:198–218.

122. James W. Pragmatism and religion. In: Gunn G, ed. *Pragmatism and Other Writings.* New York: Penguin; 1907:119–132, p. 130.

INDEX

For the benefit of digital users, indexed terms that span two pages (e.g., 52–53) may, on occasion, appear on only one of those pages.

Figures are indicated by *f* following the page number.